The Insider's Guide to Medical and Dental Schools

Bruce S. Stuart

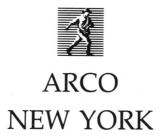

ARCO

NEW YORK

First Edition

 ARCO

Simon & Schuster, Inc.
Gulf + Western Building
One Gulf + Western Plaza
New York, NY 10023

DISTRIBUTED BY PRENTICE HALL TRADE

Manufactured in the United States of America

1 2 3 4 5 6 7 8 9 10

LIBRARY OF CONGRESS
Library of Congress Cataloging-in-Publication Data

Stuart, Bruce S., 1964-
    The insider's guide to medical and dental schools / Bruce S.
Stuart.
        p.   cm.
    ISBN 0-13-467671-8
    1. Medical colleges—United States—Directories.   2. Dental
schools—United States—Directories.   I. Title.
R735.A4S78 1988   88-19469
610'.7'1173—dc19   CIP

If you have any comments or suggestions for future editions of this book, please write to me:

Bruce S. Stuart
c/o Arco Books
Simon & Schuster Consumer Group
1 Gulf & Western Plaza
New York, New York 10023

CONTENTS

Introduction   1
Anatomy of this Book   2
  Medical/Dental School Name, Address   2
  Student Accounts   3
Admissions   3
  The Minimal Preparation   3
  GPA Statistics   4
  A Suggested Strategy for College   5
  Freshman Year   5
  Sophomore Year   5
  Junior Year   6
  Senior Year   6
  Another Piece of Advice   6
  Standardized Tests   7
Applying to Schools   7
  Advice for Dental School Applicants   8
  The Interview   8
  A Few Suggestions   9
  Recommended   10
Finances/Financial Aid   11

THE DENTAL SCHOOLS   15

  Baylor College of Dentistry   17
  Boston Univ. Goldman School of Graduate Dentistry   19
  Case Western Reserve Univ. School of Dentistry   21
  Columbia Univ. School of Dental & Oral Surgery   23
  Creighton University School of Dentistry   26
  Harvard School of Dental Medicine   28
  Indiana University School of Dentistry   31
  Loma Linda University School of Dentistry   33
  Marquette University School of Dentistry   35
  Meharry Medical College School of Dentistry   37
  N.J. Dental School Univ. of Medicine & Dentistry   39
  Northwestern University Dental School   41
  SUNY/Buffalo School of Dentistry   43
  SUNY/Stony Brook School of Dental Medicine   45
  Tufts University School of Dental Medicine   48
  University of Alabama School of Dentistry   50
  UCLA School of Dentistry   52
  UCSF School of Dentistry   55
  University of Colorado School of Dentistry   57
  Univ. of Connecticut School of Dental Medicine   59
  University of Detroit School of Dentistry   62
  University of Florida College of Dentistry   64
  University of Iowa College of Dentistry   66
  University of Kentucky College of Dentistry   68
  University of Maryland College of Dental Surgery   70

University of Michigan School of Dentistry   72
University of Minnesota School of Dentistry   74
University of Mississippi School of Dentistry   76
Univ. of Missouri/Kansas City School of Dentistry   78
University of Nebraska Lincoln College of Dentistry   80
University of North Carolina School of Dentistry   83
Univ. of Pennsylvania School of Dental Medicine   85
USC School of Dentistry   87
Univ. of Tennessee (Memphis) College of Dentistry   89
Univ. of Tx Health Ctr./San Antonio Dental School   91
University of Washington School of Dentistry   93
VCU Medical College of Virginia School of Dentistry   95

THE MEDICAL SCHOOLS   99

Albany Medical College   101
Albert Einstein College of Medicine   104
Baylor College of Medicine   107
Boston University School of Medicine   110
Bowman Gray School of Medicine   112
Brown University Program in Medicine   115
Case Western Reserve Univ. School of Medicine   117
Chicago Medical School   120
Columbia Univ. College of Physicians & Surgeons   123
Cornell University Medical School   125
Creighton University School of Medicine   128
Dartmouth Medical School   130
Duke University School of Medicine   133
Emory University School of Medicine   135
Georgetown University School of Medicine   137
Hahnemann University School of Medicine   140
Harvard Medical School   142
Jefferson Medical College   146
Johns Hopkins University School of Medicine   148
Loma Linda University School of Medicine   150
Marshall University School of Medicine   153
Mayo Medical School   155
Medical College of Ohio (Toledo)   158
Meharry Medical College   160
Mercer University School of Medicine   163
Michigan State Univ. College of Human Medicine   165
Morehouse School of Medicine   167
Mount Sinai School of Medicine   170
New York Medical College   173
New York University School of Medicine   175
Northwestern University Medical School   178
Ohio State University College of Medicine   180
Oral Roberts University School of Medicine   183
Robert Wood Johnson Medical School   185
St. Louis University School of Medicine   187
Southern Illinois University School of Medicine   190

Stanford University School of Medicine 192
SUNY/Buffalo School of Medicine 194
SUNY/Stony Brook School of Medicine 197
SUNY/Syracuse (Upstate) Medical Center 200
Temple University School of Medicine 202
Tufts University School of Medicine 205
Tulane University School of Medicine 207
Uniformed Services University of Health Science 209
University of Arizona College of Medicine 212
UC/Davis School of Medicine 214
UCLA School of Medicine 217
UC/San Diego School of Medicine 219
UCSF School of Medicine 221
University of Cincinnati College of Medicine 224
Univ. of Connecticut School of Medicine 226
University of Florida College of Medicine 229
Univ. of Hawaii John A. Burns School of Medicine 231
University of Iowa College of Medicine 233
University of Louisville School of Medicine 235
University of Maryland School of Medicine 237
University of Massachusetts Medical School 238
University of Michigan Medical School 241
University of Missouri/Columbia School of Medicine 243
University of Nevada School of Medicine 245
University of North Carolina School of Medicine 247
University of North Dakota School of Medicine 250
Univ. of Pennsylvania School of Medicine 252
University of Pittsburgh School of Medicine 254
University of Rochester School of Medicine 257
University of South Carolina School of Medicine 259
University of South Dakota School of Medicine 261
University of South Florida College of Medicine 263
University of Southern Alabama College of Medicine 265
USC School of Medicine 267
University of Tennessee College of Medicine 270
University of Texas Medical Branch at Galveston 273
University of Texas Medical School at Houston 275
University of Utah School of Medicine 277
University of Vermont College of Medicine 279
University of Wisconsin Medical School 281
West Virginia University School of Medicine 283
Wright State University School of Medicine 285
Yale University School of Medicine 287

STUDENT ACCOUNTS SECTION 291

Women 293
Woman/Older Student 296
Reverse Minority 298
Nonscience Major as an Undergraduate 299
Racial Minorities 300

Views from the Inside   300
Dental Students   300
Medical Students   301
Issues in Dental and Medical Education   302
Acquired Immune Deficiency Syndrome   302
Dental Students   303
Medical Student   303

To my parents, Vernon and Suellen Stuart, and my sister, Kim

ACKNOWLEDGMENTS

KIM D. STUART, Esq., served as the Excecutive Research Coordinator for this book. Without her tireless efforts and dedication I would not have been able to complete this project.

Dr. Robert Renner, D.D.S., gave me valuable suggestions as to the structuring of this book.
Ellen Lichtenstein, a great woman and an insightful editor.
Thank you to David Packo for providing me with two of the most meaningful quotes I have come across.
To all the medical and dental school administrators who took time out of their busy schedules and met with me although they had never heard of me before.
To Susan Maxwell and her fantastic assistant Wendy at Albany Medical College, who provided me with the GPEP Report and took the time to talk with me.
To the students who had me over at Harvard Medical School. I will never forget what you did for me and I think you guys are great!
And of course to the contributors to this book. You are the body, soul, and navigators of this project. At times I was lost and you set me in the right direction, never losing the vision of a book to help those truly in need—the applicants.
Thank you all!

TERMS USED

AADSAS American Association of Dental Schools Application Service

AAMC Association of American Medical Colleges

AAWD American Association of Women Dentists

ADA American Dental Association

AMA American Medical Association

AMCAS American Medical College Application Service

ASDC American Society of Dentistry for Children

AMSA American Medical Student Association

ASDA American Student Dental Association

Articulators Dental appartatus used to align teeth and simulate actual movement of jaw in order to check occlusion

DAT Dental Admissions Test

GPA Grade Point Average

Gunners Expression used to describe students who "shoot down" the curve (a.k.a. cut-throats)

H&Ps (Medical School term) Taking medical *Histories* and performing *Physical* examinations

Handpiece Dental equipment used to hold drill

HMO Health Maintenance Organization

JADA Journal of the American Dental Association

JAMA Journal of the American Medical Association

MCAT Medical College Admission Test

NBME National Board of Medical Examiners (a.k.a. "The Boards")

NDSL National Direct Student Loan, now called the Perkins Loan (under new federal regulations, students are independent if they (1) are 24 years of age, (2) can claim dependents other than a spouse, (3) are wards of the state or veterans, and (4) will not be claimed as dependents on their parents' next tax returns.

NIH National Institutes of Health

OB/GYN Obstetrics and Gynecology

OT Occupational Therapist

PAT Perceptual Aptitude Test (part of the DAT)

PT Physical Therapist

SES Socio-economic status [*Class* is a tainted word, whereas SES is less judgmental.]
UH University Hospital
VA Veteran's Administration Hospital

CONTRIBUTOR'S LIST

Michele Adamec
Gerald Akaka
Cary David Alberstone
Veronique T. Alcaraz
Melinda Alle
Bradley Allen
Melinda Allsbury
Raymond Amaker
Brian Anderson
Mark W. Anderson
John P. Andrews
Robert Andrews
Stephanie L. Arlis
Paul Aronowitz
Stanley H. Asensio III
Kenneth Ashley
Steve K. Aste
J. Austin
P. Kurt Bamberger
Cynthia Bamford
Michael Bard
Mary Barton
Mike Bates
Mark Beattie
Andrew J. Berens
Stephen Beveridge
Bruce L. Block
Sky Blue
Jeanne Bohrer
Barbara Bolton
Claire Borkert
Daniel Bortolotti
Michelle L. Bowman
Ann C. Bracken
Adelia Brannen

Cynthia Brattesani
Barbara Bressert
Mary Bretscher
Joe Breuner
Alan R. Brewer, D.D.S.
Jeffrey H. Brooks
Curtis Brown
Jack Brown
Jeffrey Brown
Leslie Brown
Mark Brown
Robert D. Brown, Jr.
Thomas Bruns
Joanna Buffington
R. Harrell Bullard
Mathew P. Bunyard
Brian Burgess
C. A. Burke
Catherine L. Byrne
Bill Caldwell
Jeffrey C. Cantrell
Timothy G. Caudill
Olivia Chan
Ophelia Y. Chang
Larry Chaplin
Douglas Norman Chen
Bob Clark
Tracey Clark
Lane Clower
Stephen Cobert
Todd D. Cohen
Bruce Allan Condello
Don Cork
Marlene M. Corriere
John Couk

C. Keith Cox
Kerwin C. Cox
Thomas Crabtree
Mickey E. Crosby
Rosie Marie Cruz
Salvatore R. Cutino
Eldy Dale
Amy L. Damiani
Traci Jill Dantzler
Kim Davis
Bruce DeGinder
Melissa Devalon
Angelique Devold-Amos
Elizabeth Diehl
C. Diep
Diane L. Dietzen
Kent Dodson
Roland J. Dominguez
Jon Dossett
Barry Duel
Arthur Eberly
Diane Edwards
John M. Emmett
Kristen Anne Englund
Bonnie M. Everett
Kimberly Ferguson
Eddie Finn
John Fisher
Guy D. Foulkes
Mark T. Frank
Howard Freedman
Joanne M. Fruth
Michael Furman
Corrinne M. Gallagher
Valentina Gage
Judy K. Garard
Gill Gibson
Linda Gilliam
Julie Gillis
Greg Glenn
Cary N. Goldbery
Gene M. Golding, Jr.
Brian Goldstein

William A. Greenhill
Meredith Gregory
Robert C. Griggs, M.D.
James P. Guerrieri, Jr.
Jon Gustafson
Donna J. Hagberg
Darryl Hamamoto
Sheila L. Hardee
June M. Harrison
Paul B. Hart
Elizabeth Hasslacher
Greg A. Havleka
Donald T. Hess, Jr.
Katherine M. Hickel
Dr. Joan C. Hoffman
Mark G. Hoffman
James Trent Holbrook
E. Hank Hollinger
Christopher A. Hooper
William Horton
Mary Bennett Houston
Michael Hyado
David Jacobi
Lina Jarboe
Kathleen Christie Jaroch
Jerome A. Jarosz
Jerome A. Jarus
Michael H. Jensen
Sarah Garlan Johansen
Cinde Johnston
Jay Joseph
Jaylynn Kao
Stephen R. Kaplan, M.D.
Michael Kasper
Julie Kaufman
George M. Kazakos
Greg Allan Kelley
Mike Kennedy
Sharon Kennedy
Steven P. Kiefer
Molly K. King
Anne M. Kirk
Michael K. Kluth

S. Knudsen
David Konys
Herald H. Kowa
Julie Kreager
Jack Kyle
Michael Laird
Thomas E. Langan
David J. Langer
Dennis Edward Larsen
Jim Lawson
Kass Lear
Andy Lee
David C. Lee
Insup Lee
Lisa C. Lee
Deborah A. Lenart
Gary L. LeRoy
Renne L. Lind
Joan K. Lingen
Mark W. Lingen
Madeline R. LoDucca
Angela C. Long
Brent E. Ludens
Catherine Lynch
Judy Lynch
Stephen M. Lyon
Tom Magill
Monica Makker
Debra Malley
Joseph J. Marous III
Dean G. Mastras
Daniel E. Mathews
Anne Mattson
Mary McAllister
Kathleen T.McAvoy
Julie McCann
Kenelm F. McCormick
Thomas McLoughlin
Mark H. Meacham
Sara Meloche
Julio Mendoza
Mary Mercurio
Sara Meloche

Julio Mendoza
Mary Mercu
Karen Peterson Mesner
Mona Messinger
Chris Moore
Stacey Moore
Lt. Leon E. Moores
Paul J. Mortiere
Brett L. Moses
Mike Mouri, D.D.S.
Vincent J. Murray
Jeremy S. Muscher, M.D.
Mark Mutscler
Terry L. Myers
Glenn Mylath
Brian C. Nash
Craig M. Neitzke
Amy Jo Nelson
Jan Nicoletto
Alan Novick
Chet R. Obachinski
Claire Ogatta
James Olsen
Teresa Ota
Paul Oursler
David Packo
Larry W. Parsons
Ellen Passloff
Robert Lewis Paton
Ileana R. Perez
Todd Edward Pesavento
Dr. Devereaux Peterson
John Christopher Petrozza, Jr.
Lynne C. Gilbert Pitts
Steven R. Powell
Michael A. Price
Steven Rabin
Julie Ralls
Rosa Rangel
Mark Reiber
Eric V. Reinerston, R.N.
Markus F. Renschler
Susan Rider

Kenneth B. Riley
Mike Robertson
Steven M. Robins
Nancy Edith Rodrigo
Todd Rogers
Douglas A. Rollins
Michelle Rooney
Bill Rosen
William Lee Rowland
Deborah Ellen Rudin
Daniel Saal
Robert F. Sabilis, Ph.D.
Carole Sable
Douglas T. Sakurai
Tom Scammell
Pasco W. Scarpello
Steven J. Scharpf
Donna Schwartz
Lisa B. Schwartz
Lee W. Scionti
Sanjay S. Shah
Kirk Shamley
Mark Shanfeld
June Shannon-Hughes
Raymond M. Shapiro, Ph.D.
Lynne R. Sheffler
Barbara Shotwell
Richard Silvano
Robert E. Sims
Laura N. Sinai
Karl B. Skerbeck
Jeffrey B. Smith
Kristen Smith
Mathew L. Smith
Patrick Glenn Smith
Stephen R. Smith, M.D.
David V. Snyder
Mathew A. Solberg
Jean-Louis R. Sos
Hal Sossner
Joe Spoto
Jeffrey E. Steele
Daniel C. Stewart

David W. Stroup
Larry C. Stutts
Sanjay Sunbaresan
David Sutcliffe
Mark W. Swaim
Barbara Swoyer
Rich Szumel
Roderick W. Tataryn
Jason Tauke
Jeffrey Tedrow
John K. Tidwell
Myles Tieszen
Culley Tolbert
Mark M. Zittergruen
Elise Treff
P. Glenn Tremml
Kathy A. Trumbull
Robert Uhde
Linda L. Upp
Gregg K. Vandekieft
Mark Vanderburgh
Richard Vaughn
Thomas Verborsky
Cheryl Vicari
Joseph K. P. Villagomez
Judith Wachendorf
John J. Waddell
Dean Wakham
Brett Walter
Patricia Warner
Geo. Washington
David A. Weiland
Timothy L. Weiland
Dana Weisshaar
Kimberly A. White
Jonathan W. Wilding
Deberenia E. Williams
Richard Wilmot
Michael K. Wimberly
Joseph H. L. Worrischeck
Lori Annette Wulf
Winston J. Worme
Sharon C. Worosilo

Anton Wray
Susan Wu
Daniel Wunder

Susan Yarian
Charles Young
Mark M. Zittergruen

DEBUNKING MYTHS

10 Popular Myths about Dental &

Medical Schools and the Facts

| MYTH 1 | My grade point average (GPA) and standardized test score(s) (MCAT or DAT) are really the only things that count when applying to medical and dental schools. The interview is just icing on the cake. If I have a 4.0 and perfect standardized scores I'll be accepted regardless of my interview. |

| FACT | This is a popular misconception among premeds and predents. Although GPA and test scores are considered heavily in the admissions process, the interview is also very important. As a health professional, you will be interacting with people on a continual basis, and admissions committees can only ascertain information about your social skills through the interview. At many medical and dental schools only a limited number of applicants are granted an interview. However, once you have been chosen for an interview you are generally in the same position as the other applicants. |

In short, test scores and GPAs will take an applicant only so far. After achieving a certain level, the rest of the admissions decision is determined by the interview(s). Admissions committees are looking for students who they feel are academically prepared for the rigorous course work of medical or dental school. At the same time, they are looking for mature adults who will be able to face difficult and complex decisions involving their patients' health and personal welfare.

| MYTH 2 | Dentistry is a dying profession. There are too many dentists for the number of people in our population. Go into a field with a future. |

| FACT | Dentistry is presently in a period of rapid transition. Discouragements about attending dental school are often bandied about in conversation by individuals with a limited

knowledge of the profession and its future. By the year 2000, dentistry will be more involved with aesthetics, malocclusion (orthodontics), and periodontics (disease of the supporting structures, or gums). Scientific innovations in holography (for use in dental x-rays) and laser technology (for preparing a tooth before filling it) will push dentistry to new heights. The number of students entering dental schools and the number of dentists graduating have declined, which translates into fewer dentists in the coming years. Thus, there may actually be a *shortage* of dentists for our population. Also, there will be greater emphasis placed on dentists treating more patients in underserved locations, such as rural areas, and treating a larger number of medically impaired and elderly patients.

MYTH 3 Once I get into medical school it's almost impossible to flunk out, especially in schools with Pass/Fail grading systems.

FACT This myth, often referred to as the "escalator theory" of medical school, is highly misleading and fallacious. The quantity of material covered in medical school greatly exceeds that given to students as undergraduates and at times students must put in a greater effort to achieve a "Pass" (sometimes a grade set by the school, such as 75) than was needed to get an A in college.

Do not be fooled by Pass/Fail. Although few schools wish any of their students to fail, many medical schools with this system also rank students based on the totals of the student's raw score in each class. These rankings are often used to determine what residency programs students will get at the end of the four years.

MYTH 4 All dental and medical schools are the same. You take the courses and you graduate with your D.D.S, D.M.D., or M.D. It's just that simple.

FACT It is not that simple and that was one of the major reasons for the writing of a book such as this. Each medical and dental school has different policies and different philosophies toward educating their students. Certain dental schools have their students take a separate curriculum apart from medical students; other dental schools "share" the basic sciences with the medical school. Some medical schools believe that their students should be taught by a presentation of the material by the professor; other schools have programs that require student research in order to better learn the contents of the course.

| MYTH 5 | Dental students are the ones who could not get into medical schools. Their courses are easier than medical students' courses. |

| FACT | I would not tell this one to a dental school admission's officer or to your dentist before he or she drills your teeth. This myth has become deep-rooted (pardon the pun) in our society's thinking because there is a tiny fraction of truth to it. A certain percentage of dental school students and dentists were at one time premedical students. However, most of these individuals decided not to attend medical school for various reasons, many of which have *nothing* to do with academics.

By and large, dental students really do want to attend dental schools and are generally very content with their profession. In a sense, dentistry is a specialty of medicine. Dental students simply knew what specialty they wanted and specialized earlier. As far as the curriculum being easier, this is unfounded. Often the first year of dental school is *more* difficult than the first year of medical school. This is so because medical and dental school students take the same basic sciences, but dental students also have dental courses that involve great amounts of lab work, which takes away valuable study time.

| MYTH 6 | When I get out of medical/dental school, I'm going to open up a practice by myself because it's the best way of practicing medicine/dentistry. |

| FACT | This is not entirely a myth. Solo practitioners have traditionally been fine dentists and physicians. However, for various reasons, it is becoming highly impractical to practice alone. The first reason is money. A private dental practice can easily cost $300,000 to establish, including patient lists, equipment, and other expenses such as paying dental school loans. This applies to physicians as well, due to the soaring costs of malpractice insurance. Group practices alleviate some of the costs of office space and receptionists, and many physicians and dentists find that it takes some of the pressure off them to share patients and rotate hours.

| MYTH 7 | Although you shouldn't say it in your application or tell admissions committee members, the best reason to go to medical or dental school is to make big bucks. |

FACT Medicine and dentistry will both provide you with financial security, and to many it will ensure a degree of wealth. According to the most recent AMA study available, the average income of physicians after expenses and before taxes was $113,200 [breakdown of some medical specialities: internal medicine, $101,000; surgery, $155,000; pediatrics, $77,100; obstetrics/gynecology, $122,700; psychiatrist, $80,600; anesthesiologist, $140,200* (for more about physicians' income check *Medical Economics*)]. The average net income for general practice dentists was approximately $60,000 and for specialists, $95,000.** However, for you to pursue a career in either field without an honest desire to help people through your skills is cheating not only your future profession but also your patients and yourself. No amount of money is worth being miserable in a career for at least thirty years of your life. The one indisputable reward derived by students of both medicine and dentistry is putting their learning to use by treating patients.

I have personally spoken with hundreds of dental and medical students across the country, generally after 10 P.M. After a long day of school and taking exams, they are not very enthusiastic. But when they begin talking about treating patients, their voices change. It does not take great analytical ability to realize that this is the central reward in medicine and dentistry. Money pays the bills and the loans, but it is not enough without feeling rewarded from and enjoying treating patients.

If monetary gain is your sole motivation, you would be better off pursuing another field that you are truly interested in. Chances are high that you would make a good living in that career as well. You must realize that dental and medical earnings are both beginning to level off because of Health Maintenance Organizations (HMOs) as well as increasing costs of malpractice insurance for *both* medicine and dentistry.

MYTH 8 Because of the great amount of time and committment necessary for medicine and dentistry, it is practically impossible for someone 30 or 40 years old to start dental or medical school.

FACT For those of you with this opinion, I must first refer you to the Student Accounts section of this book. Anyone who tells you that going to medical and dental school does not

---

* Socioeconomic Characteristics of Medical Practices 1986, published by the American Medical Association.

** Occupational Outlook Handbook 1986–87 Edition, published by the U.S. Department of Labor.

involve a great committment of both time and money is lying to you. But your age, economic situation, sex, religion, race, or nationality should not inhibit your decision to attend medical or dental school.

One of my primary aims for having a Student Accounts section in this book was to show potential applicants outside the "norm" that it can be done. If you have the will, there really is a way. Yes, older students may have more responsibilities, such as a spouse or family, than their younger counterparts, but they often have greater maturity and a better support network.

MYTH 9 | Medical or dental school is a lot like college with more science courses.

FACT | This is a rather myopic view of dental and medical schools. After the first two years of medical and dental school, and sometimes sooner, the student is exposed to a more hands-on type of instruction, including clinical/patient experience for dental students and rotations/patient experience for medical students.

When I began writing this book, I was advised by several medical and dental students to put a greater emphasis on the last two years of medical and dental school. They felt I should include such information as the number of babies delivered in a rotation. I thought about this for a long time and decided against it (at least in this edition of the book) for one main reason. If you think students' opinions of course difficulties are subjective, then imagine the individual variation in such figures as the number of babies delivered during one particular time of year at one particular hospital. Be aware that the similarity to the classroom/undergraduate academic experience diminishes greatly after the second year. It is also important for you to find out about clinical facilities, such as hospitals for medical school applicants and dental clinics for dental school applicants, at your prospective schools.

MYTH 10 | When I read the catalog for a medical or dental school I will find out, more or less, how much I will spend and need to budget for a year.

FACT | I have gone through every catalog of each school in this book and with very few exceptions the schools usually underestimate living expenses. You will find that medical and dental school both involve a series of hidden costs waiting to happen. To be safe, always figure on spending more rather than less for the year when anticipating funds. The "extras" may seem nominal, such as fees for lab books or supplementary texts or microscope rental fees, but these costs will add up. I have approximated costs for a single in-state (where applicable) and a single nonresident student with what students consider a reasonable amount of money for living expenses.

INTRODUCTION

I do not have to tell you that beginning something is always the hardest part. If you have ever written a paper or started reading a book (which by now I assume you have done quite often) you know that "getting into it" is the greatest challenge to be faced and met. This carries over into applying to medical and dental school as well. It's easy to begin college with the clear-cut idea that one is premed or predent. But these are only labels that by themselves are not enough to prepare you for a career in medicine or dentistry. I implore you to use your time in college wisely, to think beyond the labels, and not to become obssessed with grades. It is far more important for you to reason beyond the rote learning and attempt to understand the principles and concepts behind what is being memorized.

I must tell you that the information in this book is subjective because it has been based on the opinions of medical and dental students, administrators, and myself. I assume total responsibility for all opinions voiced in this book. Very few things you read in or out of the classroom will not be subjective; nevertheless, a warning must be made: Make certain that you use this book as *a* source and not *the* source. There is no such a thing as the perfect college or the perfect dental or medical school. What I have attempted to do in this book is to broaden your knowledge of what exists and highlight certain aspects that may be important to consider when looking at medical and dental schools.

I did not rate, rank, or give out stars for any of the schools in this book; to do so would be tantamount to saying that New York City is better than Boise, Idaho, because it has a higher population density. Some people prefer open spaces and others enjoy a more concentrated environment. Each school has its own attractions, and there may be certain things that do not interest you about particular schools. **Any** and **every** school found in this book is more than worthy of your consideration. You might notice that certain schools have been omitted. This is due to several reasons, including a lack of student participation at some schools, a less than favorable outlook at other schools (if I had nothing good to say about a school, I generally said nothing at all), and space limitations.

1

ANATOMY OF THIS BOOK

This book was designed to make it as easy as possible for you to get the information you want and need about individual medical and dental schools. The majority of the book is devoted to entries for medical and dental schools, which are grouped alphabetically in two sections. Each entry is presented in the following manner:

Medical/Dental School Name, Address

Capsule—Includes information about whether the school is public or private, its location, its age, class size, whether or not it is AADSAS (for dental schools) or AMCAS (for medical schools), exam requirements, percentage of women and minorities in the class, and average student expenditure for the first year ($ means $15,000 and under per year, $$ is $15–20,000, $$$ is $20–25,000, $$$$ is $25–30,000, $$$$$ is over $30,000 per year). Also, for medical schools: M.D.-Ph.D. and postdoctoral programs/dental specialties and NBME (National Board of Medical Examiners) requirements at each school.

Physical Environment—Living costs in the area of the school, academic and clinical facilities and their condition, the safety factor near the school, hospital sites, availability of athletic facilities, and closeness to the main campus facilities are considered in this section, among other aspects of the environs of the medical/dental school. You may not think that athletic facilities are important, particularly while you are in dental or medical school, but remember that you will be sitting for many hours in both classrooms and libraries and physical exercise is an excellent release from large doses of academics.

Academics—Includes an honest assessment by students of how much harder the work is than undergraduate science courses, grading policies, the students' opinions of their faculty, availability of student research, interesting and/or strong programs at the school, and student recommendations for courses to take before entering the school, as well as study methods once attending medical or dental school.

Financial—Gives the average dollars and cents cost for attending the school (the first year) as well as hidden costs, such as being required to buy instruments in dental schools, typical loans taken out by students, and the feasibility of working while attending the school.

Social—Tells whether or not there is time for social interaction outside the class, the activities scheduled by the school and students, and the types of students at the school.

Comments—Summarizes aspects of the school that you should consider when applying.

Student Accounts

The thoughts, feelings, and comments of selected dental and medical students across the country reflecting on being a woman, a minority, and/or a dental or medical student. The experiences of a 40-year-old woman finishing up her third year of medical school, a white medical student attending a primarily black medical school, and several other students are included. Also in this section are students' feelings about how AIDS has impacted on their medical/dental education.

ADMISSIONS

If you are worried about being accepted into medical or dental school, I have some good news for you. The competition for entrance to both medical and dental school has decreased over the last few years. I am not telling you that it is easy to gain admissions to medical or dental school, but this may be one of the best times to apply because of the decrease in the number of applicants.

Although I do address preparation along with a suggested strategy for college, this is not a "how to get into medical and dental schools" book. To put it bluntly: Nobody can take your tests for you and/or ultimately decide whether or not you should be a physician or dentist but you. One book (or even several) of advice is not the way to get into medical or dental school. You can take suggestions from what you read, but once again, *you* must decide your plan of action with help from parents, your dentist or physician(s), prehealth advisors, and even "Getting into————" books.

As you may have already realized by turning the pages, there are *no* admissions statistics given with each school. However, I feel that because admissions is a major concern of most premedical and predental students, I should address this aspect of medical and dental education in this book.

The Minimal Preparation

There are certain basic premed/predent requirements for each school, usually including the following courses:

1 year of biology (some schools require one or two extra semesters)
1 year of general chemistry

1 year of organic chemistry

1 year of physics

1 year of college English (recommended: at least one semester of writing)

1 year of mathematics (recommended: one semester of statistics)

This book gives suggestions for other courses that students should consider taking as undergraduates before entering medical or dental school. There are some overlapping courses recommended and some students believe that the minimal requirements are "just fine."

Remember that any familarity you have with a basic science in medical or dental school, such as biochemistry, histology (a.k.a. microscopic anatomy), gross anatomy, physiology, genetics, microbiology, and pharmacology, will make the courses that much easier. Although it is not an easy process, students may be able to place out of certain basic sciences, particularly biochemistry, if they have a strong enough background from their college course(s). This greatly lessens the first-year course load, which by any standard will be heavy.

GPA Statistics

There are several reasons why I did not publish the omnipresent (and thus inferred to be omnipotent) GPAs for dental and medical schools. The first reason is because, as I stated earlier, this is not an admissions book. The second is because these figures are often misleading. Anyone with a basic knowledge of statistics knows that numbers can be made to "look good." This does not mean that schools are giving factually incorrect information, but that the numbers can be taken out of context.

A major source of confusion arises when somewhat outdated statistics are used that may not reflect major changes in GPA that occurred over a short period, such as the dramatic drop-off in GPA of several private dental schools. The final reason is that these figures only reflect the mean GPA of the students who were accepted and are *not* indicative of student A's chance of getting accepted to medical or dental school from Huskerdue University with a 3.7 as opposed to Student B coming out of Johns Hopkins with a 3.4.

I'm not saying not to look at the numbers (you will find that the majority of medical schools in this country have a 3.5 mean GPA plus or minus .2 and most dental schools, with the exception of a few schools with smaller classes, have a mean GPA of 3.0 plus or minus .2), but please use the figures you are given by schools and books as a loose guideline—not as a definitive marker of your chances for admissions. They are not.

A Suggested Strategy for College

Freshman Year: **Relax**.   This is the year of the "weed out" courses. This tends to be the hardest year because the introductory science courses are designed to "size down" the number of premedical and predental students at the school. Do not overload with several science courses unless you have an exemplary science background from high school. Rather, take a lighter load first semester with perhaps one or two introductory science classes and or a math class (statistics is very useful).

You should use this time to get adjusted to the difficulty of college courses as compared to the high school or Advanced Placement classes you took in high school. Stop in and visit your prehealth advisor and let him or her know that you are interested in dentistry or medicine. The longer he or she knows you, the better he or she will be able to guide your course decisions and later write a letter of recommendation.

If for some reason this year does not proceed as you had hoped academically and you still want to attend medical or dental school, do not give up! **Never** allow one or two courses to terminate something that you really desire. However, if you feel that you are beating your head against the wall after taking further science courses (such as over that summer) you might consider other options.

Sophomore Year: **Broaden your horizons**.   Take as many courses as you are interested in taking, as well as two science classes per semester (chemistry and biology are good choices).   At this time, you should begin thinking about a major.   A word about this, there is **no** preference given to science majors, so that if you like the humanities you should pursue this along with your premedical/predental courses. In keeping with medical and dental student recommendations, you might keep in mind that a course in computers, business, and/or economics should prove very useful.

Use the summer after this year to work in a capacity related to your chosen interest. Premeds might work at hospitals, with area physicians, or at nursing homes. Predents should be involved in an area that fosters their manual dexterity. This will be a tremendous advantage when you enter dental school where lab projects tend to occupy a longer period of time for those with poorer manual ability. You do not have to work for a general dentist or a dental specialist (though this would be a very good experience) to gain manual dexterity. Sculpture, drawing, or painting, as well as model-making, are excellent ways to fine-tune your fingers.

Junior Year: **Major decisions. A busy year**. Now is the time to start making up your mind about whether you are interested in dentistry or medicine. You should have chosen a major that you feel comfortable with (and enjoy) regardless of the subject. Music and philsophy majors have been accepted to dental and medical schools along with their biochemistry and biology counterparts.

By now, you can handle a larger load of science courses, so you might consider taking biochemistry if it is not part of your major. If possible, you should consider conducting research in an area of your interest, such as research seminars or writing a thesis in your field of study. You can do research in biochemistry or sociology, but what is most important is that you are actively interested in learning about a discipline *beyond* what is written in your required texts. Advances in both medicine and dentistry depend on research and the ability to integrate and piece together new information into the matrices of previously existing knowledge.

During this year, you should consider your options (described later) for standardized exams. The sooner you take them, the less pressure you will have if you need the chance to retake the DAT or MCAT. This year also involves obtaining recommendations. Try to get recommendations from professors who know you very well, such as professors from small seminars, faculty advisors, and/or research supervisors. You should begin your AMCAS/AADSAS application as early as possible during this year and obtain application forms from nonmember schools to which you wish to apply.

Senior Year: **Travel light**. This year will, it is hoped, involve a number of medical or dental school interviews, When planning your course load, you should realize that your time will be consumed by travel. In other words, lighten your academic load.

Another Piece of Advice

When choosing courses during the academic year, try to take the strongest science courses you can handle. If you are worried about getting a poor or marginal grade in an upper-level course, audit it. At least you will have the exposure to the subject matter under your belt before entering dental or medical school. Although grade point averages are important, other criteria are used in considering applicants, among them the personal interview and what you have done with your time in college besides studying for exams.

Standardized Tests

Just when you thought taking tests was all over, here they are again. And this time you often have one or maybe two tries to do your best, making each try a high-pressure experience. You have three ways to approach the MCAT or DAT.

1. Conduct your own review by going over your notes and old books. This plan of action is for the highly self-motivated individuals who either do not want to spend money for a prep-course or feel there is no need for such an investment. If you are going to study on your own, make certain you start early enough to organize the material you're reviewing (usually done by the test prep book or course).

2. Buy a test prep review book and drill yourself using the tests in the book. Again, this requires much self-motivation, but if you have come this far, you certainly have the drive to review on your own. A word to the wise: *Always* check the publication date of the book. Outdated test prep books (anything two or more years old) are a waste of your valuable time and money.

3. Take a test prep course. I highly recommend this option if you have the money (between $500 and $600) and the time before the exam (generally four to six weeks), and if you need a little shove now and then to get motivated. There are numerous such prep courses, but it is my opinion from experience with students and my own familiarity with such courses that Stanley Kaplan is the best test prep course offered for both the DAT (especially good visual aids to help you with the Perceptual Aptitude Test) or the MCAT.

APPLYING TO SCHOOLS

It has often been said that an applicant should apply to as many schools as he or she can afford. This is not a wise strategy. If you do not have any intention of attending a medical or dental school why throw away the application fee and possibly the expenses, including transportation and lodging, involved with travelling for an interview? You should apply to the state schools of medicine or dentistry in your home state not only because of their lower tuition but also because you have a better chance of being admitted to schools that must accept a large percentage of in-state residents by law. Then, consider the other schools and choose from the ones that most interest you. There is nothing wrong with applying to a large number of schools, but make sure you have chosen the correct "group."

Advice for Dental School Applicants

In light of the recent decision to phase out Georgetown School of Dentistry, which was preceded by Emory and Oral Roberts dental schools, applicants must be careful not only when applying but also when choosing dental schools. No one can tell you if and when there will be another or several dental school closings. To be safe, consider the following aspects of each school:

1. Is it private or public? Private schools generally have a riskier economic situation because of fewer (if any) state subsidies.
2. Has the school, particularly private dental schools, cut down on the size of its class in anticipation or in response to a smaller applicant pool? (This is generally a good sign.)
3. Have there been cutbacks in faculty or full-time staff at the school? (This may be a sign of the anticipation of a closing)

It is best not to be paranoid. Although it is an unpleasant experience, students whose schools close will generally be able to graduate from these schools or be placed in other dental schools rather than being pushed out on "the street." But you must exercise caution and careful judgment when applying to and choosing among dental schools.

The Interview

This is an important component of the medical/dental school admissions process. You must be willing to "package yourself." Make a list of your best qualities. What sets you apart from other applicants? Try to get a list of interview questions from your prehealth advisor. If you cannot, sit down and make them up. Pretend you are the admissions officer. Sometimes the interviewer will have your academic record on hand. At other interviews (called "blind" interviews), the interviewer will not be provided with your grades, standardized test score(s), essay, and recommendations.

Obvious questions you might ask are: Why are you interested in dentistry/medicine? How did you like your college/university? What do you think about socialized medicine/shopping mall dentistry? What is the thing you like least/most about yourself? Have you conducted your own research? What are your interests/hobbies? How do they tie in with dentistry/medicine? What do you think about the rising cost of a medical/dental education? What impact do you think

AIDS has had on our society? On the health professions? What area of dentistry/medicine would you like to specialize in? (The list is endless!) After you have gone over the list, practice answering the questions with a good friend or parent, giving the "interviewer" the opportunity to add other questions that you might not have thought of.

A Few Interview Suggestions

Interview Clothes: After you've been accepted you can wear shorts and a T-shirt, but during the interview you must project the proper image. Wear something conservative that also makes a statement such as a grey flannel/navy suit with a vibrant colored tie for men and a sedate suit with skirt or a dress for women (not too much makeup or excessive jewelry). Remember: Most of your interviewers will be in their mid-forties and fifties.

Neatness: Everyone should try to present a neat appearance. Dental applicants should be especially careful to make sure their fingernails are very clean and well manicured. After all, would you want someone's dirty fingernails in your mouth?

What not to do: Do not act pompous or overbearing with your interviewer. Try to impress but not overwhelm or self-aggrandize your achievements to the point of nausea. Do not bluff the answer to a question you know absolutely nothing about. It is better to say "I am not aware of such and such. Could you elaborate on your question?" and have your interviewer explain his or her question rather than to make a complete fool of yourself.

For Dental Applicants: Chalk-carving tests are given at a few dental schools as part of the admissions process (especially for applicants with poor or marginal PAT scores) during the day the interview(s) is held. Do not worry about breaking the chalk. Many students who break their chalk are accepted. What is important is that you know which schools have the test and practice carving a piece of chalk at your leisure. [HINT: A piece of paper towel (if provided) can make a big difference in smoothing over rough surfaces!]

Before the Interview: Read some of the latest medical/dental journals or books. Below are some of the more widely read and highly respected publications about medicine, dentistry, and advances in science, as well as some sources of informative entertainment.

Recommended

For advances in medicine and dentistry:

Journal of American Dental Association (JADA)

Journal of American Medical Association (JAMA)

The New England Journal of Medicine

The New York Times (particularly Tuesday's *Science Times*)

For history/interesting information/admissions statistics

Admission Requirements of U.S. and Canadian Dental Schools 1988–89 by the American Association of Dental Schools.

Dental Education in the United States and Canada: A Report to the Carnegie Foundation for the Advancement of Teaching by William John Geis. The Carnegie Foundation, 1926.

Five Thousand Years of Medicine by Gerhard Nenzmer. Taplinger, 1972.

The Flexner Report(s) by Abraham Flexner. The Carnegie Foundation, 1910.

The Language of Medicine: Its Evolution, Structure, and Dynamics by John H. Dirckx. Harper & Row, 1976.

Love, Medicine, and Miracles: Lessons Learned about Self-healing from a Surgeon's Experience with Exceptional Patients by Bernie Seigal. Harper & Row, 1976.

Medical Acronyms and Abbreviations by Marilyn Fuller Delong. Medical Economics Book, 1985.

Medicine in America; Historical Essays by Richard Shyrock. John Hopkins Press, 1966.

The Miracle Finders: The Stories Behind the Most Important Breakthroughs of Modern Medicine by Donald B. Robinson. David McKay Co., 1976.

"Physicians for the 21st Century," *Journal of Medical Education* Vol. 59, No. 11, November 1984 (also known as the GPEP Report)

Sympathy and Science by Regina Markell Morantz-Sanchez. Oxford University Press, 1985.

They All Laughed at Christopher Columbus: Tales of Medicine and the Art of Discovery by Gerald Weissman. Times Books, 1987.

For entertainment:

The House of God by Samuel Shem, M.D. (at times the most hilarious and moving of books; definitely takes your mind off worrying about your interviews)

"St. Elsewhere" (Marcus Welby, M.D. could have learned a lot from this show! Look for it in reruns.)

"M*A*S*H" (both the television show reruns and the motion picture)

An apology to dental applicants: The media has continued to portray dentists in a negative (and often brutal) light. Hopefully, future books, television shows, and movies will more accurately portray this very honorable and respected profession.

A Final Word: Relax. The most important thing for you to have in the interview is not the fact that you are a Nobel Laureate or a Rhodes Scholar (though it might help). What you need most is to believe in yourself. If you have that, you've got everything you need. Good luck!

FINANCES/FINANCIAL AID

A major deterrent to medical and dental education is the exorbitant cost of attending these schools. There is a financial section included with each school entry which estimates the average cost for a single, in-state student to attend the school being discussed. When anticipating costs, it is always smart to inflate the cost, this way you will have too much allotted rather than too little.

With most dental and medical schools costing $15,000 a year or more, it is only reasonable to expect that the majority of medical and dental students will take out some type of loan. Many schools offer grants, but by and large, middle-income students must pay their expenses with a combination of parental/spousal contributions, loans, grants, and/or working. As far as working while attending medical or dental school, I have asked students at each school to comment on its feasibility and on which academic years it is most possible.

The following are a list of the most common federal loans for dental and medical students. An asterisk means if you need a loan, this one is recommended.

*1. *Guaranteed Student Loan (GSL)* A very valuable loan that most health professional students take out during the course of their education. This loan is made by credit unions, savings and loan associations, or banks. Dental and medical students may borrow up to $7500 a year for the full period of graduate study, which cannot exceed a total amount of $54,750 including GSL loans made to the same student as an undergraduate. The interest on this loan is 8 percent for all new loans and 7 or 9 percent for students with previous GSLs. Each time a loan check is issued, a 5-percent origination fee is deducted and passed on to the federal government to help reduce the cost of subsidizing the loans.

You must begin repaying a GSL 9 to 12 months after leaving school for 7-percent loans and 6 months after leaving for 8- or 9-percent loans. For further information write to (or phone): Department of Education, Office of Student Financial Assistance, 400 Maryland Avenue, S.W., Room 4050-ROB 3, Washington, D.C. 20202, (202) 732-3154.

*2. *National Direct Student Loan (NDSL)* This loan, now called the Perkins loan, has a limit of $18,000 for graduate students. The loan carries a 5-percent interest charge, which starts 9 months after graduation for new borrowers and 6 months after for previous borrowers. For further information write to (or phone) Department of Education, Office of Student Financial Assistance, 400 Maryland Avenue, S.W., Room 4050-ROB 3, Washington, D.C. 20202, (202) 732-3154.

3. *Health Alliances Loan (HEAL)* This is the most expensive loan of the group warned against by many students and schools because of its variable interest rates (3 percent above the Treasury bill rounded to the next highest ⅛ of 1 percent). It was once called the "loan of last resorts." Regretfully, it is becoming a frequently used loan because of the increasing cost of medical and dental schools. Under this loan, students may borrow up to $20,000 a year for four years for a maximum of $80,000. You have 33 years to pay back the loan but do not allow time to fool you. This is a very expensive loan even at the current lower interest rates. Take out as much money as you can on other loan programs before applying for this one. For further information write to: Chief, HEAL Branch, Room 839, 5600 Fishers Lane, Rockville, Maryland 20857.

*4. *PLUS and SLS Loans* These loans are part of the GSL program and allow parents to borrow up to $4000 a year for a maximum of $20,000 (beyond the limits set by GSL). You do not have to pay an origination fee, as you do with GSLs, but a state guarantee agency can charge you up to 3 percent of the loan principal, which will be deducted from each loan payment. The maximum interest for this loan is 12 percent, and you must begin paying it back within 60 days after completing your dental/medical full-time education. For further information write to (or phone): Department of Education, Office of Student Financial Assistance, 400 Maryland Avenue, S.W., Room 4050-ROB 3, Washington, D.C. 20202, (202) 732-3154

These are some of the federal loans available. If you want more information you can write away to the following address for *The Student Guide—Five Federal Financial Aid Programs*: Student Aid Programs, J-8, Pueblo, Colorado 81009-0015.

There are also several loans and scholarships for minority students and women. I have listed a few:

Links, Inc., Scholarship: This is for minority students who are residents of the Boston area and have been accepted at an accredited dental or medical school. For more information write to: Links, Inc., Scholarship Program, 129 St. Paul's St., Brookline, Massachusetts 02146.

Fellowships for Native Americans You may apply if you are at least one-fourth American Indian, Eskimo, or Aleut; enrolled as a member of a tribe, band, or group recognized by the Bureau of Indian Affairs, enrolled in an accredited college or university; and in financial need. For more information write to: American Indian Scholarship, Inc., 5106 Grand Avenue, N.E., Albuquerque, New Mexico 87108.

American Association of University Women (AAUW) This is a one-year stipend for the final year of either medical or dental school in the amount of $3500 to $8000. For more information write to: AAUW Educational Foundation Programs, 2410 Virginia Avenue, N.W., Washington, D.C. 20037.

Clairol Loving Care Scholarships Eligibility is open to women at least 30 years old who will complete their program of study within 2 years of the award date. Awards range from $500 to $1000. For more information write to: Scholarships, BPW Foundation, 2012 Massachusetts Avenue, N.W., Washington, D.C. 20036.

Grace Le Gendre Fellowships These are open to female graduate students who are New York State residents. Financial need and scholastic ability, as well as good health, are factors considered. Awards of $1000 are given annually and are renewable. For more information write to: BPW Clubs of New York State, 125 Mayro Building, Utica, New York 13501.

THE
DENTAL
SCHOOLS

BAYLOR
College of Dentistry
3302 Gaston Avenue / Dallas, Texas 75246

LOCATION: Urban/Big City

AGE OF SCHOOL: 83 Years

CONTROL: Private (With state subsidy)

AADSAS **MEMBER:** No

CLASS SIZE: 100

PERCENT WOMEN IN CLASS: 33

PERCENT MINORITIES IN CLASS: 10

AVERAGE STUDENT EXPENDITURE: $ (In-state); $$$ (Nonresident)

POSTDOCTORAL PROGRAMS: Yes; endodontics, oral and maxillofacial surgery, orthodontics, pedodontics, periodontics, prosthodontics; also, combined programs with undergraduate schools

---

PHYSICAL ENVIRONMENT

Although Baylor College of Dentistry is located in the medical center, the school's building is a separate entity, along with a seminar building, a medical library, and a multilevel parking garage. One of Baylor's strongest features is the school's outstanding and innovative clinical facilities. The operatories are structured in such a manner as to make the student feel as if he or she is practicing in an actual dental office. The basic sciences facilities are very good and the school has access to a new gym.

The area around the dental school is relatively safe. Finding reasonably priced housing near the school does not present a problem for students; the cost of a one-bedroom apartment in the area of the school is between $300 and $350 per month. Dallas provides students with numerous opportunities for shopping, theater, and nightclubs. The library is considered "excellent, particularly for [video and audio] cassette players with instructional tapes and microfiche viewing machines."

ACADEMICS

Baylor dental students recommend taking a wide spectrum of courses, "particularly courses that you always wanted to take but never got around to," including biochemistry, English, art ("something to do with aesthetics and proportions which is becoming more and more important in dentistry"), computers, and business management courses. The courses here are "demanding and fun at the same time, because you really enjoy learning all of the information. There's just so much of it!" Students begin formally working with patients during their second year. They find this arrangement to be good because they feel they have mastered enough basic and clinical sciences before working on a patient.

Competition for grades is "there but not fierce." Students wishing to enter specialty programs generally work hardest and increase the competition in the classes. Going over all old tests, studying with a partner, attending all lectures, and copious note-taking are considered good ways of preparing for tests. Physiology, biochemistry, and histology are considered among the hardest courses. The faculty are considered very knowledgeable and reasonably accessible when "truly needed by the student." Endodontics, Periodontics, and Oral Surgery are thought to be among the strongest departments at this school.

FINANCIAL

The difference in tuition between in-staters and nonresidents at this school is very large, with the total for the first year for residents costing $12,500 and for nonresidents, $20,000. Students buy their instruments for a total cost of about $8500, with payment occurring over the first two years. Thus, the last two years are much less expensive. Working is not recommended until after the first year when there are some jobs available through the school and the community.

SOCIAL LIFE

School sponsored parties at this dental school are few, but students hold keg parties and other functions during the course of the year. There are several older students at this school and a significant number of out-of-staters.

COMMENTS: Baylor is an excellent value for Texas residents but is far more expensive for nonresidents. The school has the advantage of excellent clinical facilities, a good location, and a strong faculty.

BOSTON UNIVERSITY
Goldman School of Graduate Dentistry
100 East Newton Street   /   Boston, Massachusetts 02118

LOCATION: Urban/Big City

AGE OF SCHOOL: 13 Years

CONTROL: Private

AADSAS **MEMBER:**   Yes

CLASS SIZE: 52

PERCENT WOMEN IN CLASS: 28

PERCENT MINORITIES IN CLASS: 35

AVERAGE STUDENT EXPENDITURE: $$$$$ (Both In-state and nonresident)

POSTDOCTORAL PROGRAMS: Yes—available in most dental specialities

PHYSICAL ENVIRONMENT

Boston University (BU) dental school is located in its own modern building across the way from University Hospital and the medical school. The area immediately surrounding the dental school is safe, but outside of this perimeter the going gets a little tougher. As with most Boston schools, students find living expenses to be high because of housing. The average cost of a one-bedroom apartment is about $600 per month. Most students choose to live away from the area of the dental school and commute. Mass transit in Boston is relatively reliable and the school is within a ten-minute walk of the bus and the "T."

The dental school has very modern facilities because the school is relatively new. Operatories are clean and labs are well maintained at this school. The school is removed from the undergraduate campus and has limited accessibility to some athletic facilities. However, the undergraduate campus facilities are accessible across town by car.

ACADEMICS

BU dental school has had a problem for several years in that the students did not "feel like dental students" for the first year of school. They rarely were inside the dental school and were instead taking the same basic sciences courses as their medical school counterparts. Because BU is a young school that is also open to changes, the administration was recently able to add more dentistry-oriented courses in the first year.

Students find their course work far more challenging than their undergraduate science courses because of the amount of memorization and reading required. It is strongly recommended that prospective students take biochemistry, and business management/ economics courses, as well as art courses fostering manual dexterity, before entering.

Faculty are considered very knowledgeable and willing to assist— more so in the dental courses than in the medical school courses. Competition for grades is definitely present due to both a letter grade system for evaluation and increased competition for specialty programs among students. It is recommended that students use both note cards and study groups when studying for exams. Most departments are considered very strong, particularly Restorative Dentistry. One major benefit from this school is the constellation of outstanding programs in graduate dentistry to which several students choose to apply after completing their four years at BU. Endodontics, Periodontics, and Aesthetic Dentistry are considered very strong at this school.

FINANCIAL

Whenever you ask students at BU dental school about the school they will not fail to mention the exorbitant cost. Conservative estimates for a year of study range from $35,000 to $40,000. Students buy their instruments for approximately $5300, with most (about $4000) due during the second year and the rest the first year. How do students cope with the high cost of studying here? One student answered with a very serious face: "You take out loans. And then when you're done with those loans you take out more. If I didn't think this place was worth the money I certainly wouldn't be taking out all these loans." Students here are taking out every loan offered to dental students, including HEAL loans.

SOCIAL LIFE

Attending school in the Boston area affords BU dental students several opportunities for socializing and sight-seeing. Cambridge, Quincy Market, and countless restaurants and museums are favorite spots. There are some school-sponsored parties as well as get-togethers organized by students.

COMMENTS: Students here are very happy about the inclusion of more dental school courses earlier on in their education. However, without exception, all students here feel overburdened by the cost of attending. BU—Goldman School of Graduate Dentistry is a fine dental program, especially if cost is not a major concern to you.

CASE WESTERN RESERVE UNIVERSITY
School of Dentistry
2123 Abington Road / Cleveland, Ohio 44106

LOCATION: Urban/Big City

AGE OF SCHOOL: 96 Years

CONTROL: Private

AADSAS **MEMBER:** Yes

SIZE OF CLASS: 80

PERCENT WOMEN IN CLASS: 30

PERCENT MINORITIES IN CLASS: 15

AVERAGE STUDENT EXPENDITURE: $$$ (Both in-state and nonresident)

POSTDOCTORAL PROGRAMS: Yes—oral surgery, orthodontics, periodontics, and pedodontics; also, accelerated 7-year programs available in conjunction with several Ohio colleges

PHYSICAL ENVIRONMENT

The Case Western Reserve School of Dentistry is situated in the Health Sciences Center. One student comments about the clinical and basic sciences facilities: "This school has every piece of modern dental equipment imaginable. The lab areas are very well spread out and the clinic is well run and well equipped." Case is located in a reasonably safe neighborhood which borders both "good and bad" sections of Cleveland. Athletic facilities at the main campus and numerous places to "escape from school," such as the museum of art, are within easy walking distance.

Many students choose to live in off-campus housing which costs about $250 to $300 per month for a one-bedroom apartment. It is not necessary to have a car because of a very reliable mass-transit system. Besides, there's a parking shortage on campus.

ACADEMICS

Many students here feel that Case's program was one of the major drawing cards for this dental school. Both basic sciences and clinical courses are taught simultaneously, with more basic sciences the first two years and more clinical work the last two years. This gives students the opportunity to draw correlations between what they are learning in the classroom and in the clinic. It is recommended that predental students take biochemistry ("You might be able to place out"), courses fostering manual dexterity (such as sculpting and drawing), and business management.

During their fourth year, students are able to work in areas of their own interest if they have completed all the basic requirements. Seniors also work in a "private practice–type" environment under the supervision of a dentist. Competition for good grades is not intense among students and they go out of their way to help one another. According to one student, "Doing well is accomplished by a systematic and organized review of the material and getting hold of any old tests if humanly possible. . . . Also, use upperclassmen as references. Most of the time they'll be willing to help if you need it."

The faculty is spoken very highly of. Students praise faculty members both for their accessibility and for their well-structured lectures. There are numerous opportunities for student research, particularly during the fourth year. Orthodontics, Restorative Dentistry, and Periodontics are considered very strong departments at this school.

FINANCIAL

Case will cost the average first-year dental student about $21,000. Students buy their instruments for about $6300, with the majority of payment occurring over the first two years; so the third and fourth year will cost considerably less money. Most students take out a combination of federal loans, and the school offers a few scholarships to students who demonstrate extraordinary financial need. Students advise aginst working the first year, but say that after that it is feasible and there are several jobs in the area that pay well.

SOCIAL LIFE

Students find that there is time for a social life. One student adds, "Professors are good about making sure you don't have too many exams all on the same day." There is a good mixture of students from many different backgrounds, including a significant number of older students. Both the school and students sponsor parties.

COMMENTS: Case has the major advantage of a very good curriculum and a caring faculty and adminstration. Students here enjoy the school's location of their school because of its proximity to athletic, cultural, and shopping facilities.

COLUMBIA UNIVERSITY
School of Dental and Oral Surgery
630 West 168 Street / New York, New York 10032

LOCATION: Urban/Big City

AGE OF SCHOOL: 136 Years

CONTROL: Private

AADSAS **MEMBER:** Yes

CLASS SIZE: 60

PERCENT WOMEN IN CLASS: 37

PERCENT MINORITIES IN CLASS: 33

AVERAGE STUDENT EXPENDITURE: $$$$ (Both in-state and nonresident)

POSTDOCTORAL PROGRAMS: Yes—available in conjunction with numerous dental specialties; also, combined D.D.S.-Masters of Public Health Administration available

PHYSICAL ENVIRONMENT

Columbia University School of Dental and Oral Surgery is located within the Columbia Presbyterian Medical Center. The school's labs are very adequate, and the student clinics, which have been renovated within the last 10 years, are well laid out and spacious. The inside of Columbia is much less intimidating than the surrounding area, which, although it is undergoing a slight rejuvenation, is dismal and not in the most scenic of areas. Nonetheless, most students say that it is relatively safe. A subway ride will get students to the main campus facilities, which are located several miles away.

Finding housing near the school seems to be little problem. There are several housing facilities for students. These include Bard Hall which is being renovated and costs about $3100 per year; The Georgian, which has suites and kitchenettes and ranges from $2700 to $2900 per year; and The Haven Tower Apartments, which has one-, two-, and three-bedroom apartments. Students prefer living in the latter (if they can obtain housing there) because they can share three-bedroom apartments for about $400 per month. Students recommend living in student housing because it costs less than most off-campus accomodations.

ACADEMICS

Some dental schools have been known to lower their academic standards, particularly in years when the applicant pool has declined. Columbia has attempted, and for the most part succeeded, in maintaining its very good reputation by cutting the size of its class and making a coscientious effort to accommodate its students with financial aid packages as much as possible. Competition for good grades is intense for dental students, and the course work is very demanding. Dental students here take their basic sciences with the medical school, giving them the chance to learn from one of the top basic sciences faculties in the country. It is recommended that students take courses in molecular genetics, biochemistry, Spanish, and histology before attending this school.

Pharmacology and biochemistry are among the more difficult basic sciences, and students strongly recommend keeping up with the course work. Student research opportunities are phenomenal. Research is encouraged due to the presence of a research-oriented faculty (both clinical and basic sciences) and an honors research society. The faculty are outstanding in their field, and the student/faculty ratio is excellent in the dental clinics.

Many students selected this school based on its reputation and faculty. As a result of its location, Columbia attracts a wide variety of patients and cases. Columbia has an excellent record for placing its students in postgraduate and general practice residency (GPR) programs.

FINANCIAL

Columbia will cost first-year students about $30,000. Students buy and rent their instruments for approximately $6000, which is paid for over a four-year period. Each student is given a financial aid work sheet, and every effort is made to assemble a suitable financial aid package for each accepted applicant. Working is recommended only during the last two years, and there are well-paying jobs in the hospital.

SOCIAL LIFE

There is not a great deal of time for a very active social life, particularly the first two years, although the cultural opportunities in New York City are limitless. Some class parties and happy hours are held by students and the school. Columbia attracts dental students from almost every background imaginable. What they all have in common are their strong academic abilities and competitiveness.

COMMENTS: Columbia is a very fine dental school with an outstanding record for placing its graduates in GPR and postgraduate programs (which many students opt for). The basic science instruction is among the best in the nation because students take their courses with the medical school. There is no question that you will receive a topnotch dental education at this school. As far as the location (Washington Heights) is concerned, it is very urban and, as mentioned earlier, somewhat dismal. However, other New York attractions—such as shows, night clubs, museums, and health clubs—are a subway ride away.

CREIGHTON UNIVERSITY
School of Dentistry
2500 California Street / Omaha, Nebraska 68178

LOCATION: Urban/Medium-Sized City

AGE OF SCHOOL: 110 Years

CONTROL: Private (Religious affiliation: Jesuit)

AADSAS **MEMBER:** Yes

SIZE OF CLASS: 75

PERCENT WOMEN IN CLASS: 11

PERCENT MINORITIES IN CLASS: 3

AVERAGE STUDENT EXPENDITURE: $ (Resident of pact states); $$ (Nonresident of pact states)

POSTDOCTORAL PROGRAMS: No

PHYSICAL ENVIRONMENT

Creighton University dental school is located on the Health Sciences Campus and is housed in a modern building constructed in the early 1970s. The university is the smallest in the United States to have a full complement of health sciences, which include Creighton Medical School and Creighton School of Dentistry. The dental school building is an impressive structure with spacious clinical areas and technologically advanced equipment.

Students here remark about the school's library, which one student calls "a comfortable learning environment with outstanding resources." The school shares facilities with other health sciences schools and is affiliated with numerous hospitals. The area around the school is considered safe, and finding housing does not appear to a problem. The average cost for a one-bedroom apartment near the school is between $300 and $350 per month.

ACADEMICS

Students recommend taking biochemistry, histology, and "any other basic sciences which may help you the first year," along with courses fostering manual dexterity, such as sculpting and drawing. Formal experience with patients begins during the later half of the second year. Students find this amenable because, as one says, ". . . I feel it's very important to know what you're doing before you start working on patients. It makes the learning experience more meaningful if you can relate what you learned to what you're doing in the clinic." Competition among students for good grades is very much present, although students are not cut throat.

Creighton offers interesting clinical experiences, such as a summer program in Latin America and the opportunity to work in a geriatric center as well as in several hospitals. The faculty are regarded highly and show deep concern for students and their learning interests. There are numerous opportunities for student research under the supervision of a faculty member. Endodontics and Restorative Dentistry are considered very strong departments at this school.

Several states with dental schools of their own have pacts with Creighton, including Idaho, New Mexico, North Dakota, Utah, and Wyoming. Students from these states receive a substantial discount in their tuition. Idaho students may enroll in IDEP (Idaho Dental Education Program) and can enter either Creighton or Idaho University their freshman year; Utah residents may enroll in RDEP (Regional Dental Education Program) giving them the option of entering either the University of Utah or Creighton their freshman year.

FINANCIAL

Creighton will cost first-year students a total of approximately $16,000. Students from pact states will pay less because of lowered tuition. Students buy their instruments for a total of $4500, with payment occurring during the first two years, which makes these years more expenisve than the junior and senior years. Most students take out financial aid in the form of GSLs, and Creighton offers some scholarships and loan programs of its own. Students warn against working but say it is possible on a limited basis after the first year.

SOCIAL LIFE

Creighton has an adequate social life, and students remark that the "school's religious philosophy adds a healthy atmosphere to the class." There are many gatherings planned by students and the school, including parties and recreational sports. The school attracts a small number of women and minority students.

COMMENTS: Creighton dental students often comment about the "philosophy" (stated by the school) at this school. For those who have strong religious convictions, particularly Jesuits, this may definitely be the place. The school has excellent extramural internship programs and very good clinical facilities.

HARVARD SCHOOL OF DENTAL MEDICINE
188 Longwood Avenue / Boston, Massachusetts 02115

LOCATION: Urban/Big City

AGE OF SCHOOL: 121 Years

CONTROL: Private

AADSAS **MEMBER:** Yes

CLASS SIZE: 25

PERCENT WOMEN IN CLASS: 50

PERCENT MINORITIES IN CLASS: 10

AVERAGE STUDENT EXPENDITURE: $$$$ (Both in-state and nonresident)

POSTDOCTORAL PROGRAMS: Yes—numerous programs available in conjunction with several dental specialties

PHYSICAL ENVIRONMENT

Harvard School of Dental Medicine borders on the Harvard Medical School quadrangle and is adjacent to the Harvard School of Public Health. The dental facilities are primarily contained in a large brick building that combines its long history (first university dental school in the country) with modern and up-to-date facilities. There are three clinics: one for faculty, one for students who are in their first four years, and another for students who are in their fifth year. The operatories are very new and spread out, with several being partitioned.

The school is located away from the main undergraduate campus; however, students have easy access to a gym which is within a five-minute walk. Several first-year dental students choose to live in Vanderbilt Hall, which is shared with medical students. Costs are between $280 and $360 per month, and students who return their housing application before the deadline can rest assured that they will be able to live there.

ACADEMICS

For the first two years, Harvard School of Dental Medicine students presently take the same classes as medical students who are in the Classic Curriculum at Harvard Medical School. However, it is important to note that in the 1987–88 school year, and thereafter, the Classic Curriculum will have certain courses like the Oliver Wendell Holmes Society, which employs case histories and independent research. Thus, dental students will also be taught with this method. Furthermore, if the Harvard Medical School in future years decides to use this method of teaching for all its students, dental students will also be taught entirely by this method for their first two years.

Another unique aspect of Harvard is the fact that students attend for five, rather than four, years. During the fifth year, students conduct research and write a thesis. Some students use this fifth year to begin their specialty education in such fields as orthodontics and periodontics. However, this year is not applicable to oral surgery residencies. Students are very enthusiastic about having the opportunity to spend more time conducting research than they might have had the chance to do at four-year dental schools.

Competition for grades is not intense, due in part to the Honors/Pass/Fail grading system used at Harvard. Students recommend studying in small groups. Students here also have the opportunity to train at some of the top hospitals in Boston and the country, including Massachusetts General Hospital. Faculty are generally experts in their field and, for the most part, easily accessible to students. Implantology is on the "cutting edge" of dentistry at this school. Periodontics and Endodontics are considered very strong departments by students.

FINANCIAL

Harvard School of Dental Medicine will cost about $30,000 per year for single students their first year. Some dental instruments are bought by students and others rented, costing approximately $7000, which is payable during the second, third, and fourth year of school. There are numerous financial aid packages offered by the school. Students concerned about the fifth year of education should be aware that many fifth-year students are able to get grants and/or stipends for their research and many are already enrolled in specialty programs which pay part of their way. Fifth-year students also have their own clinic in which they treat patients (and are paid). This can be used to make up the expenses of this year.

SOCIAL LIFE

Harvard offers its students the opportunities of Cambridge, Boston, and many historic sites. Students have many social gatherings during the year. The class itself is very small and relatively "cliquey." Students are very bright and concerned about dentistry and its future. Many of the students have research interests and pursue them during their fifth year at Harvard. You will find few general practitioners graduating fom this school, although every year certain students accept associateships. The vast majority of students are interested in specialties and/or teaching at a dental school.

COMMENTS: A major deterrent for students considering this school is the additional year and its expense. If you are interested in either specializing and/or conducting research while at dental school, then do *not* be dissuaded by the fifth year. As mentioned above, there are ways provided by the school, in addition to loans, that can help to alleviate the cost of the last year. Harvard School of Dental Medicine offers its students boundless opportunities for research, as well as outstanding basic science and clinical training. The school also offers a large number of postdoctoral programs, including orthodontics and endodontics.

INDIANA UNIVERSITY
School of Dentistry
1121 W. Michigan Street / Indianapolis, Indiana 46202

LOCATION: Urban/Big City

AGE OF SCHOOL: 63 Years

CONTROL: Public/State

AADSAS **MEMBER:** Yes

CLASS SIZE: 115

PERCENT WOMEN IN CLASS: 21

PERCENT MINORITIES IN CLASS: 15

AVERAGE STUDENT EXPENDITURE: $(In-state); $$ (Nonresident)

POSTDOCTORAL PROGRAMS: Yes—M.S. and M.S.D. programs available in most departments.

PHYSICAL ENVIRONMENT

The dental school is interesting architecturally because it is made up of an older building that has a more modern addition. The classroom facilities are modern and provide up-to-date audiovisual equipment. Some of the clinics have older equipment, such as for crowns and bridges. Plans for renovation are currently being considered.

The dental school is located three minutes away from the nationally known Natatorium, which houses swimming pools and athletic equipment. The school is fairly centered between the medical center complex and the undergraduate schools.

The school is located in a large city, and the area immediately surrounding the school is not considered a good place to live. However, students who need housing can find apartments for about $300 per month in the general vicinity of the dental school.

ACADEMICS

Students mention faculty most often when talking about the school's programs. "They really care about you knowing what you're doing and make you feel like an individual rather than just another student." Students find that there is some competition for grades

("That is to be expected"), and letter grades are used to evaluate their work during the first three years. "It really gets a lot better after the first three years," adds one student. The curriculum eases students into the clinic gradually, and at the same time the faculty try to correlate what is learned in the classroom with what is experienced in the clinic. It is recommended that students get old exams when possible, study in groups, and take extensive notes on readings.

Fourth-year students have numerous opportunities for pursuing their own interests in dentistry by choosing from over 200 extramural settings, such as private dentists, local clinics, and state and federal institutions. A project is required for graduation, in the form of either an essay/thesis or table clinic. Students here recommend taking biochemistry, histology, and carving and/or model-making before attending this school. Endodontics, Periodontics, and Oral Surgery are all considered very strong departments.

FINANCIAL

Indiana will cost a total of $12,500 for in-state first-year students and $16,500 for nonresidents. Students both buy and rent their instruments for a total of $5000, with payment primarily during the first two years. The financial aid office at this school is considered very good by students, and there are some scholarships and loans given out each year. Most students advise against working, particularly during the first year.

SOCIAL LIFE

Indiana students feel that there is an adequate social life at their dental school. Most activities, such as parties at students' apartments or houses, are initiated by students. There are a significant number of nonresident students accepted and attending this school.

COMMENTS: The faculty is excellent at this school. In-state students, as well as nonresidents who want a quality dental education in a school with very good clinical facilities, should definitely apply here.

LOMA LINDA UNIVERSITY
School of Dentistry
Loma Linda, California 92350

LOCATION: Suburban/Small Town

CONTROL: Private (Religious affiliation: Seventh-Day Adventist)

AADSAS **MEMBER:** Yes

CLASS SIZE: 70

PERCENT WOMEN IN CLASS: 25

PERCENT MINORITIES IN CLASS: 32

AVERAGE STUDENT EXPENDITURE: $$$ (Both in-state and nonresident)

POSTDOCTORAL PROGRAMS: Yes—M.S. available in conjunction with several dental specialties

PHYSICAL ENVIRONMENT

Loma Linda Universtiy (LLU) School of Dentistry is made up of both old and new buildings that blend surprisingly well. The buildings used for the first-year basic sciences are between 50 and 60 years old. The dental school and medical center are modern and are located on an attractive smaller campus.

The campus is small, making all facilities easily accessible and within a five minute walk. There are tennis courts and a gym, although there is no swimming pool. A new activities center and a pool are planned to be completed next year.

The dental facilities are up to date, and whenever anything breaks, it is repaired immediately. The clinic area is not crowded and is a pleasant place to see patients.

Finding housing is not a problem at Loma Linda dental school. Students can live in on-campus dorms or choose from one of the many available rentals in the area of the school. Living conditions on campus are tight, but off-campus is fine. The median price for apartments is between $250 and $500 per month. The area around the school is suburban and relatively safe.

ACADEMICS

"Students should be prepared to study much harder than at their undergraduate school," advises one woman about attending Loma Linda dental school. Take the "fun courses" you will never have time to take after you enter dental school. Also recommended are histology, biochemistry, and "definitely a few business courses." Tests are mostly multiple choice at this school, and there is not much competition among the class for grades. Biochemistry, pharmacology, and histology are among the hardest courses encountered by students. Endodontics, Restorative Dentistry, and Oral Surgery are highly recommended departments at this school. There is an adequate supply of patients for students to treat in the clinic.

It is important to keep up with material and to learn to memorize. A good suggestion for succeeding here is to not procrastinate and to reward yourself by taking time to "play" by participating in intramural sports, or some other sort of exercise. The students speak very highly of faculty and say that "They [faculty] . . . are 100% supportive and treat us fairly and as equals." There are many opportunities for student research, ranging from basic sciences to clinically applied research. Students study about five hours a day during the first two years.

FINANCIAL

Loma Linda dental students expect the first year of school to cost approximately $20,000. Students purchase their instruments for about $6400, with the bulk of payment occurring over the first and second years of study. Most students have loans, and it is possible to work at the university during the second and fourth years (the school will not allow students to work during the first year, with a few exceptions) and in the surrounding neighborhood.

SOCIAL LIFE

Loma Linda is a religiously affiliated dental school. Students here comment that "LLU has a strong Christian base that is also shown through its faculty and staff." Students are honest and say, "This school isn't for everybody. Most people are devout Christians and those that aren't lead a similar lifestyle. This is not a 'party' school though people do 'party', but keep it *very* quiet." Some of the "shocks to the system" include prayer before class, a minimum requirement of religious courses, and chapel at least once a week. There are parties, beach trips, and talent programs organized by students and the school. Students here are religious and individualistic and very positive about their school.

COMMENTS: Loma Linda has very good facilities, a fine location, and a strong faculty. One additional thing that applicants should take into consideration is the school's strong religious philosophy and highly devout student body. As one man says, "For some students, they will think Loma Linda was designed with them in mind. However, other students can find that the school is just not for them. You must consider this school while taking into consideration your own personality makeup."

MARQUETTE UNIVERSITY
School of Dentistry
604 N. 16th Street / Milwaukee, Wisconsin 53233

LOCATION: Urban/Big City

AGE OF SCHOOL: 81 Years

CONTROL: Private

AADSAS **MEMBER:** Yes

CLASS SIZE: 115

PERCENT WOMEN IN CLASS: 22

PERCENT MINORITIES IN CLASS: 43

AVERAGE STUDENT EXPENDITURE: $$ (Both in-state and nonresident)

POSTDOCTORAL PROGRAMS: Yes—endodontics, orthodontics, fixed and removeable prosthodontics, and dental materials.

PHYSICAL ENVIRONMENT

Marquette University School of Dentistry is housed in an older gothic-style building that has been remodelled inside. The school is across the street from the recreational center and a short walk from the student union. The school's clinical facilities are newly renovated and have the latest dental equipment, including panarex and modern x-ray equipment for orthodontic evaluation.

Marquette is located in downtown Milwaukee, which is a larger metropolitan area with several opportunities for shopping, theater, and recreational activities. It is not difficult to find housing in the area of the school. Housing is more expensive closer to the school but becomes cheaper about a mile out. The average one-bedroom apartment is between $250 and $300 per month. Some students live in fraternity houses and pay very inexpensive rent ($60 per month, all included). The area around the school is considered relatively safe. Students might want to bring a car if they wish to travel away from campus frequently.

ACADEMICS

The work load is slightly more difficult than undergraduate science courses. One student recommends that predents take neuroanatomy, histology, and as much anatomy as possible, as well as biochemistry, immunology, and genetics. He felt that taking these courses "freed me up to spend more time on my lab courses. Also, the base of knowledge I had coming in made it easier to learn much more of the material presented in class above what I already knew."

Competition for good grades is not intense because most classes use a straight scale, so it is possible for all students to do well. Anatomy, microbiology, and neuroanatomy are among the hardest basic sciences courses taken by students. Repetition is considered the best study skill because the material is not difficult and should be easily managed if reviewed frequently.

The faculty are spoken of highly at Marquette, and according to one student, "They are one of Marquette's greatest assets." They are very personable and help students whenever it is necessary. Research is encouraged by the faculty and there are several opportunities for student research.

FINANCIAL

Marquette will cost between $20,000 and $22,000 for the first year of study. Students buy their instruments for a total of about $8500, with payments primarily over the first two years. Most students take out loans, primarily GSL loans with HEALs as a last resort. There are many opportunities to work both through the school and in the

Milwaukee area, but it is recommended that students (especially in the first years) work only during breaks and summer vacation.

SOCIAL LIFE

There are plenty of chances to socialize at Marquette School of Dentistry, including fraternity parties (there are two fraternities), class parties, intramural sports, several clubs, and student faculty-mixers.

COMMENTS: Marquette's faculty are among its best features. Students here find the location of the school to be ideal. The clinic is well run and has the latest technological equipment.

MEHARRY MEDICAL COLLEGE
School of Dentistry
Nashville, Tennessee 37208

LOCATION: Small Town

AGE OF SCHOOL: 102 Years

CONTROL: Private

AADSAS **MEMBER:** Yes

SIZE OF CLASS: 46

PERCENT WOMEN IN CLASS: 52

PERCENT MINORITIES IN CLASS: 90

AVERAGE STUDENT EXPENDITURE: $ (Both in-state and nonresident)

POSTDOCTORAL PROGRAMS: No

PHYSICAL ENVIRONMENT

Meharry Medical College School of Dentistry is housed in a new building located near the other Meharry health science colleges. The clinical facilities have been renovated recently and are in very good condition. Operatories are grouped according to dental speciality, and there is a special section of operatories that the faculty use for demonstrations. Students comment that the area around the school is questionable and that students should take safety precautions when walking at night. Students find that the dental schools' proximity to other health sciences colleges is convenient because there is greater access to learning resources. There are several audiovisual aids, as well as computer learning programs, accessible to students.

It is not difficult to find housing near the school. The average one-bedroom apartment costs between $250 and $300 per month. Meharry has on-campus housing facilities including Dorothy Brown Hall, which houses 70 women ($121 for a double and $133 for a single per month), and the Student-Faculty Towers, an apartment complex that houses both faculty, staff, and students (between $175 and $250 per month). Most students choose to live in either dormitories or apartments. It is recommended but "not necessary" to bring a car to campus.

ACADEMICS

Meharry uses a committee system approach to learning. Students take basic sciences along with some preclinical courses their first year and gradually move into the clinic. It is strongly recommended that students take microbiology, biochemistry, social sciences, and a course in speed reading before attending this dental school. Competition for good grades is not apparent, and students go out of their way to help one another. Mnemonics, study partners, and outlining the material presented are recommended for success at this school.

The faculty are considered very good both in teaching and helping students with difficulties. Meharry provides free academic counseling and professional study habit analysis to students. There are opportunities for student research, but the student must take the initiative.

FINANCIAL

The first year at this school will cost students approximately $15,000. Students buy their instruments for about $7500, with the bulk of payment made during the second year. Most students take out loans of some sort and the financial aid office is considered very good. There is a work/study program for students who wish to have work while enrolled at the school.

SOCIAL LIFE

Students find limited opportunities for social interaction due to the heavy amount of work. There are some social events, such as class parties, sponsored both by the school and students. The class is easygoing and bright, and members get along very well.

COMMENTS: Meharry is a sound dental school with an excellent faculty, very good facilities, and a vibrant study body. The school has a mission to provide quality health care to underserved areas, and by all accounts it is succeeding in its mission and with graduating quality dentists.

NEW JERSEY DENTAL SCHOOL
University of Medicine and Dentistry
100 Bergen Street / Newark, New Jersey 07103

LOCATION: Big City

AGE OF SCHOOL: 18 Years

CONTROL: Public/State

AADSAS **MEMBER:** Yes

CLASS SIZE: 88

PERCENT WOMEN IN CLASS: 30

PERCENT MINORITIES IN CLASS: 20

AVERAGE STUDENT EXPENDITURE: $ (In-state); $$ (Nonresident)

POSTDOCTORAL PROGRAMS: Yes—endodontics, oral surgery, orthodontics, pedodontics, periodontics, prosthodontics, and general practice residencies

---

PHYSICAL ENVIRONMENT

New Jersey Dental School is comprised of modern and well-cared-for buildings. The school is situated in a relatively unsafe area, but there is an escort service. All athletic and campus facilities are within easy walking distance (a walk across the street). The clinical facilities are modern (only eight years old), and recently the chairs were replaced in one of the four clinics.

The cost for a one-bedroom apartment is between $300 and $350 per month. Because most students do not live near the school, having a car is considered almost a necessity. Most students elect to share houses in order to keep their living costs down.

ACADEMICS

The course work at this school is rigorous, and students strongly recommend taking biochemistry and microbiology before entering. Competition for good grades and "gunners" are present in the classes, and there is an increasing push toward general practice residencies and specializing after graduation.

An effective method of studying includes studying alone and getting together afterward with a group of students to discuss the material. Physiology and microbiology are among the hardest courses for students. Endodontics, Periodontics, and Oral Surgery are considered to be excellent departments.

The faculty are helpful and understanding of students' needs and problems. There is a strong emphasis placed on family practice dentistry. Research opportunities are especially good during the summer, at which time there is a Summer Research Fellowship program for interested students.

FINANCIAL

The cost of New Jersey Dental School for a resident runs about $11,000 for the year as opposed to $13,500 for nonresidents. Students rent their drill, handpieces, and articulators, which helps keep costs down. They purchase their instruments for approximately $3200, with the majority of the payment over the first year. The school has a work/study program, and students feel that working is quite possible while enrolled at this school. Most students take advantage of loans and any scholarships for which they are eligible.

SOCIAL LIFE

There are many social events scheduled for students. The dental school has student dinners, outings to baseball games, picnics, and trips. The students here are highly competitive, but they are still willing to help one another when the going gets tough.

COMMENTS: Newark, New Jersey, may not be an ideal location for learning dentistry, but the instruction and opportunities for research at this school are excellent. The clinical facilities are also very good. New Jersey Dental School is a good school for both New Jersey residents and nonresidents to consider.

NORTHWESTERN UNIVERSITY
Dental School
311 East Chicago Avenue / Chicago, Illinois 60611

LOCATION: Urban/Big City

AGE OF SCHOOL: 97 Years

CONTROL: Private

AADSAS **MEMBER:** Yes

CLASS SIZE: 95

PERCENT WOMEN IN CLASS: 30

PERCENT MINORITIES IN CLASS: 32

AVERAGE STUDENT EXPENDITURE: $$$$ (Both in-state and nonresident)

POSTDOCTORAL PROGRAMS: Yes—available in conjunction with numerous dental specialties

PHYSICAL ENVIRONMENT

Northwestern University Dental School is located on Chicago's Gold Coast and is housed in a very modern building. The school is located two blocks from campus housing. Facilities such as a gym, a pool, racquetball courts, squash courts, and a cafeteria are located inside the individual dormitories. Everything the student needs is encompassed in a two- to three-block span.

The facilities within the dental school are quite good, and the school is well equipped with advanced technological equipment. The freshman and sophomore technique labs are located in the Ward Building, which was donated by Montgomery Ward. These facilities are much older and not as modern as the clinic. However, there is adequate space and they serve their purpose.

As stated earlier, the campus is located on the Gold Coast, a few blocks away from the Magnificent Mile. It's a beautiful area for shopping, sightseeing, sunbathing, and swimming, sailing, and rowing. It is a few blocks from Lake Michigan. Above all, the school is located in a relatively safe area.

Most students who live near the school live in the on-campus dormitories, which are spacious, comfortable, and much cheaper than comparable housing in the city. Student housing runs about $4500 per year, which includes room ($3200) and board ($1300). A studio apartment that is not affiliated with the school will cost about $5000 for the year, not including eating expenses.

ACADEMICS

The difficulty level of courses is comparable to undergraduate courses. However, students find that the number of courses taken at one time and the rapidity with which they must learn material causes the work to be much heavier. Anatomy, biochemistry, and physiology are recommended for predents considering this school. It is also wise to take course work that will improve hand skills and visual acuity, such as painting, sculpting, and architectural drafting.

Competition for grades is considered intense because several classes work their grading scale based on the grades of the top five students in the class. The faculty are well known for their research achievements. One student comments, "The faculty here are great. Some will approach you and others you must approach. But, all are very friendly and willing to help you." There are opportunities to do research, but most students do not think there is ample time for this until junior year. Pathology, removable prosthodontics, microbiology, and operative dentistry are among the hardest courses. Removable Prosthodontics, Fixed Prosthodontics, and Oral Diagnosis are considered very strong departments at this school.

It is recommended that students take advantage of the note service in order to prepare for classes ahead of time. Obtaining old exams is another key to succeeding on exams.

FINANCIAL

Northwestern is an expensive dental school, and most students here feel this is the school's biggest (if only) drawback. Students rent the bulk of their dental instruments for a four-year total of about $3000.

A conservative estimate for the first year at this school is about $30,000. Most students have loans, and the school does provide job opportunities for people who need "spending money." Students can work from the first year in research jobs or jobs at the dormitories, but it is strongly recommended to avoid working at all costs. Not only is the school work demanding, but the free time you have is necessary in order to "cool down" from the day's work.

SOCIAL LIFE

The dormitories offer social interaction with medical and law students, who all share the cafeteria and dorm facilities. There are also three dental fraternities that are very socially active. The school itself sponsors some social functions such as wine and cheese parties. Students here have diverse backgrounds; many are from foreign countries. One thing that practically all students agree upon is that the class is very competitive.

COMMENTS: Northwestern Dental School is a solid dental school with excellent facilities and clinical faculty. The one drawback, as previously mentioned, is the very high cost of attending this school.

SUNY/BUFFALO
School of Dentistry
325 Squire Hall   /   Buffalo, New York 14214

LOCATION: Suburban/Medium-Sized City

AGE OF SCHOOL: 96 Years

CONTROL: Public/State

AADSAS **MEMBER:** Yes

SIZE OF CLASS: 87

PERCENT WOMEN IN CLASS: 20

PERCENT MINORITIES IN CLASS: N/A

AVERAGE STUDENT EXPENDITURE: $ (In-state); $$ (Nonresident)

POSTDOCTORAL PROGRAMS: Yes—available in conjunction with numerous dental specialties.

PHYSICAL ENVIRONMENT

"If there was a crowding problem before, there certainly isn't one now!" These are the words of a dental student who is commenting about the recent construction of Squire Hall. This modern and attractive facility, completed only a year ago, has more than doubled the school's capacity for clinical equipment and instruction. It is located on the South Campus near the outskirts of Buffalo. The area around the school is considered safe. Students recommend bringing a car to "get around town." The school is about a 15-minute drive from campus athletic facilities.

Buffalo has numerous hospital affiliations as well as satellite clinics, and the locations give students a reasonably good mixture of patients from different backgrounds. Most students prefer to live in off-campus housing, and the cost of a one-bedroom apartment in the area of the school is about $300 per month. Some students elect to invest in homes for the four years they are there. The school is near many cultural and shopping areas, reachable by both car and mass transit.

ACADEMICS

Competition for good grades (A/B/C/D/F) is rather intense. Says one student, "This is a great place if you're academically prepared before you get here. If not you might find you have some trouble up ahead." Students strongly recommend taking as many basic sciences courses as possible, including biochemistry, physiology, and some form of human anatomy. There are numerous research opportunities available to students, particularly during the summer when research fellowships are offered.

The curriculum is diagonal and begins first year with mostly basic sciences and a clinical course in preventive dentistry. The basic sciences decrease and there is an increase in the amount of clinical work until the fourth year, when all work is in the clinic. Although students find that the clinical faculty "have the edge" over the basic sciences instructors, both groups of faculty are spoken well of as far as ability to convey information is concerned.

It is recommended that students review old tests, take notes on readings, and attend all lectures for academic success. A considerable percentage of the classes are interested in specializing after graduating from this school.

FINANCIAL

Buffalo will cost first year in-state students approximately $12,000 and nonresidents, $16,000. Students do not buy the bulk of their instruments, so the cost is cut down to a total of $3000 paid in equal portions over the four years. Students advise against working while attending this school because of the heavy work load. Almost all students take out a loan of some sort; many have GSLs and there are some Regents Scholarships available to residents who meet the academic and financial qualifications.

SOCIAL LIFE

There are some parties organized by the school, but by and large most are organized by the students themselves. The class is a mixture of students primarily from New York, with a good number from both downstate and upstate.

COMMENTS: Buffalo has the advantages of brand-new facilities, an outstanding faculty actively involved in research, and a highly motivated and caring student body. New York State students should definitely consider applying to this dental school.

SUNY/STONY BROOK
School of Dental Medicine
Stony Brook / New York 11794

LOCATION: Suburban

AGE OF SCHOOL: 20 Years

CONTROL: Public/State

AADSAS **MEMBER:** Yes

CLASS SIZE: 27

PERCENT WOMEN IN CLASS: 45

PERCENT MINORITIES IN CLASS: 25

AVERAGE STUDENT EXPENDITURE: $ (In-state) (Nonresidents generally are not accepted.)

POSTDOCTORAL PROGRAMS: No

PHYSICAL ENVIRONMENT

Stony Brook School of Dental Medicine is located on the main campus of SUNY/Stony Brook. The school is made up of relatively modern square-shaped glass buildings. Stony Brook dental school is close to campus facilities, which are accessible by a campus shuttle. There are shopping malls and restaurants within driving distance of Stony Brook. almost all students have a car because of the great distances traveled getting around Long Island. However, there is a bus service from outside the University Hospital, where first and second year students take basic sciences with medical students. Stony Brook is located in a very safe suburban area.

It is not difficult to locate housing at Stony Brook if you are there early enough. Many first-year students opt for on-campus housing at Stage XVI Apartments (also known as Chapin). Chapin is very inexpensive, and some students try to live there all four years for this reason. Most, however, move out (quite willingly) after their first year. Housing costs around Stony Brook are relatively high, ranging from $450 to $550 per month for a one-bedroom apartment. Many students escape these high costs by living in nearby areas such as Port Jefferson and Setauket, where they share houses and apartments. Sharing houses is very common at Stony Brook. The clinical facilities at Stony Brook are excellent with modern operatories and clean work areas.

ACADEMICS

Stony Brook School of Dental Medicine can easily be considered one of the strongest dental schools in the country. It has a rigorous program that integrates basic sciences, dental courses, and lab work. This is done to let students get into the clinic during their first year. It is a difficult program because of the lab work and information required of first-year students. Students at this school recommend taking biochemistry before entering because placing out (which few students actually do) lightens your work load first semester considerably. Other recommendations are for time management courses and psychology.

Tests are graded fairly. Although professors at this school are very demanding, they are also very accessible and "bend over backwards" to help students who need assistance in any course. Faculty at the dental school will even stay after hours to help students before tests. Pediatric Dentistry, Periodontics, and Restorative Dentistry are all excellent and highly recommended departments at Stony Brook.

FINANCIAL

Stony Brook allows students to rent almost all their equipment for a total of approximately $2200, spaced out equally over the four years, except for handpieces, which cost $200 the first year. Everything else is rented and practically all other supplies are provided at no cost to the student. There are no out-of-state students at Stony Brook at this time; costs for in-state students are about $15,000 per year total. Most students take out GSL loans, with a few taking out HEAL loans. Work opportunities, such as tutoring students, are provided. However, the intensity of the first year makes outside working all but impossible.

SOCIAL LIFE

Stony Brook School of Dental Medicine has a very small class. This is both good and bad. Although students here are provided with far more individual attention than at most dental schools, the small class size tends to cause cliques to develop. Students know what each other student says within minutes of it being said. However, certain classes are very tightly knit. It is important for students at this school to work together because there are so few of them. Students are encouraged to this end by school-organized wine and cheese functions and two recently formed dental fraternities. The fact that there are two fraternities at a school this small says something about the industry of the students here. There are several parties at the beginning of the year and after major exams.

COMMENTS: You will find more than a few students at Stony Brook had also been accepted to the Harvard School of Dental Medicine. Stony Brook is a young school that over a very short period of time has built itself a reputation as one of the leading schools of dental medicine in the nation. This is due in part to the innovative faculty and administrators at Stony Brook and largely to the outstanding students which have been attracted to this school since its inception. If you are a New York State resident considering dental schools, this is one of your best bets.

TUFTS UNIVERSITY
School of Dental Medicine
One Kneeland Street / Boston, Massachusetts 02111

LOCATION: Urban/Big City

AGE OF SCHOOL: 120 Years

CONTROL: Private

AADSAS **MEMBER:** Yes

CLASS SIZE: 125

PERCENT WOMEN IN CLASS: 37

PERCENT MINORITIES IN CLASS: 20

AVERAGE STUDENT EXPENDITURE: $$$$ (Both in-state and nonresident)

POSTDOCTORAL PROGRAMS: Yes—available in almost all the dental specialties

PHYSICAL ENVIRONMENT

Tufts School of Dental Medicine is housed in a white, 10-story sky-scraper that looks like an office building. The school borders China Town and the "Red Light" district, which is rapidly eroding. It is safe to walk alone during the daytime and with groups at night. Tufts School of Dental Medicine is not located on the Medford Campus where there are several athletic facilities. However, there are nearby athletic clubs and a multitude of restaurants, and cultural and shopping areas within easy walking distance of the school.

Tufts School of Dental Medicine has maximized its space and has phenomenal dental clinic facilities. Operatories and equipment are state of the art, and because of the school's excellent reputation for delivering quality dental care, several patients choose to go to Tufts dental clinics. The student labs are slightly crowded but are adequate.

There are no student dorms, and housing around the area of the dental school runs from $600 to $800 per month for an apartment. Many students opt for housing that is farther away or share apartments to cut down on costs. It is not necessary, and at times impractical, to have a car while at this school because getting a parking space is difficult and mass transit is very good.

ACADEMICS

Tufts dental students do not take classes together with the medical school students. Some students say they like this better because the curriculum is centered around dental concerns and topics rather than being crammed into a section of a course designed primarily for medical students. Competition for good grades is, as one student puts it, "More than apparent. Students here are very competitive for general practice residencies as well as specialty programs." The school employs letter grading for most courses.

Students recommend taking computer and business courses in addition to basic predent requirements. One woman says, "Whether we like it or not, dentistry is not only delivering quality health care, but there is a business end to it also." Students find pathology to be among the hardest courses. Endodontics, Periodontics, and Restorative Dentistry are considered to be very strong departments. It is stressed that reviewing notes, as well as continual studying with some cramming before tests, is the key to academic success.

FINANCIAL

Tufts School of Dental Medicine will cost the average single student between $25,000 and $30,000 for the first year. Students at this school buy their instruments for approximately $4300, with payment occurring primarily over the first two years. The majority of students take out as many loans as possible, and the school gives some grants. When asked about the cost of attending, one woman said, "You get what you pay for."

SOCIAL LIFE

Talking with students one feels that they have active social lives relative to other dental students. There are several parties sponsored by the school and by student groups and organizations, of which there are quite a few. One man commented, "Why live your life in a book? There's more to an education than just cramming for tests."

COMMENTS: When United States dental schools are mentioned, Tufts usually comes to mind. It was, and still is, one of the better and more progressive schools of dentistry in the nation. However, like almost all private dental schools, the escalating costs of attending have deterred some students from attending. Regardless of this fact, if you attend Tufts, you will leave having gained outstanding clinical experience.

UNIVERSITY OF ALABAMA
School of Dentistry
SDB Box 16 University Station / Birmingham, Alabama 35294

LOCATION: Urban/Big City

AGE OF SCHOOL: 43 Years

CONTROL: State/Public

CLASS SIZE: 55

AADSAS **MEMBER:** Yes

PERCENT WOMEN IN CLASS: 25

PERCENT MINORITIES IN CLASS: 5

AVERAGE STUDENT EXPENDITURE: $ (Both in-state and nonresident)

POSTDOCTORAL PROGRAMS: Yes—dental public health, endodontics, oral pathology, oral surgery, orthodontics, pediatric dentistry, periodontics, prosthodontics, and general practice residencies.

PHYSICAL ENVIRONMENT

University of Alabama School of Dentistry is housed in an older structure that has been enlarged (five-story addition) and that was renovated in the mid-1970s. The school is right on the Birmingham Campus of the University of Alabama and is located in a downtown area that students say is reasonably safe. The clinical and lab areas at this school are excellent, with the clinics set up for four-handed dentistry. Athletic facilities, including a pool, weight equipment, and racquetball courts, are housed in the gym that is about eight blocks from the school.

Housing around a five-mile radius of the dental school is not difficult to find and is less expensive than many other major cities in Alabama. A one-bedroom apartment costs between $250 and $350 per month. It is suggested that students might want to bring a car in order to get around Birmingham, although mass transit is available.

ACADEMICS

Students at this school find the work to be both rigorous and demanding. One student says, "Tests that I took in dental school that covered three to four weeks of material often included more material than final exams for the science courses that I took as an undergraduate." It is helpful to have a background in biochemistry as well as human anatomy before matriculating, and students recommend taking such humanities courses as English, psychology, and communications. Competition for good grades is very much present the first year but quiets down considerably after that.

Students believe that studying alone is a good method for succeeding along with taking notes on the texts and learning how to cram. Alabama has one of the five National Institutes of Dental Research, which students feel attracts a very capable and at times intimidating faculty. However, students find that once they take the initiative, the professors are more than willing to go over material with them. There are abundant opportunities for student research, and the class is broken down into smaller groups of students under the tutelage of a member of the faculty. Students selected this school primarily for its excellent reputation and location. Periodontics, Oral surgery, and Endodontics are considered to be very good departments at this school.

FINANCIAL

Alabama School of Dentistry has the advantage of *very* low in-state and nonresident tuition compared to other dental schools. The total cost of the first year for residents is $10,000 and for nonresidents, $11,200. Students buy their instruments for about $5100, with the bulk of payment occurring over the first two years of study. Working while in school is strongly discouraged for the first two years because of the heavy work load. Most students take out loans, particularly the Alabama State Dental Scholarship Program (available to Alabama residents), during the course of the four years.

SOCIAL LIFE

Social activities at the school include barbecues, parties, and dances, although some students here feel the social life is "nothing to write home about." A significant number of nonresident students are accepted to and attend this school each year. All agree that their class is made up of hard-working, fun-loving individuals who enjoy what they're doing and will help other students.

COMMENTS: Alabama School of Dentistry offers several advantages to its students, including a very reasonable cost for attending, small class size for more individual attention, good clinical and basic science facilities, and an extremely well-qualified faculty. The teaching philospophy here is that dentists are physicians of the mouth rather than technicians. In the words of one student, "I would highly recommend the school to someone who is looking for an excellent education and who is not afraid of working hard."

UNIVERSITY OF CALIFORNIA/LOS ANGELES
School of Dentistry
Center for Health Sciences / Los Angeles, California 90024

LOCATION: Urban/Big City

AGE OF SCHOOL: 28 Years

CONTROL: Public/State

AADSAS **MEMBER:** Yes

CLASS SIZE: 88

PERCENT WOMEN IN CLASS: 33

PERCENT MINORITIES IN CLASS: 7

AVERAGE STUDENT EXPENDITURE: $ (Both in-state and nonresident)

POSTDOCTORAL PROGRAMS: Yes—available in numerous dental specialties

---

PHYSICAL ENVIRONMENT

UCLA is a large campus with a beautiful mixture of architectural styles. The medical center, which is located on the edge of the campus, is very large and easy to get lost in. There are beautiful botanical gardens located close to the dental school. The dental school itself is about 25 years old and is a 10-minute walk from the campus gym, bookstore, and financial aid office. Although this distance may not seem far, one student points out that it is just out of reach for noon time sports activities and running errands for financial aid checks. However, the Center for Health Sciences is immediately next to Westwood, a social hub of Los Angeles containing shops and boutiques and restaurants.

The facilities within the dental school are described as looking used but in very good condition. New equipment has been installed, including 100 new dental chairs this past year. One complaint shared by several students is the amount of space for students in the clinic. This problem should be rectified by a reduction in the size of future classes. The dental school is part of the campus, and one feels this although the city itself is only a block away.

UCLA dental school students bemoan the high cost of living in the area surrounding their school. Searching for housing requires time, energy, and money. However, the areas surrounding UCLA, Beverly Hills, Bel Aire, Brentwood, and Westwood, are very safe to walk in at night. Housing, as mentioned previously, is very expensive surrounding the dental school, with a one-bedroom apartment costing between $550 and $750 per month and a two-bedroom apartment going for between $800 and $1250 per month. Sharing rooms in apartments is seen by most as the key to keeping housing costs down. Apartments are by far the most common form of housing, however, 10 percent of the class takes advantage of family student housing which has a 12-month wait.

ACADEMICS

The course load is ". . . massive and demanding, particularly the second year." (This comes from students who scored among the top in the nation on the DAT) Students spend most of their time taking basic sciences during their first year and then are given a great many lab classes in their second year. They begin formally working with patients during the second semester of the second year. Course recommendations before entering stress such disciplines as child behavior, education, psychology, and extracurricular activities that prepare you to interact effectively with people from different backgrounds. Knowledge of molecular biology, physiology, and biochemistry would greatly ease the course load.

Students all agree that the Pass/Nonpass grading system at UCLA dental school is among its best features. Students are able to do "special reports" if they wish to "go for grades." The hardest courses encountered by students are pharmacology, removable prosthedontics, and preclinical courses in fixed prosthodontics as well as oral pathology. Students' methods for studying emphasize developing sound study skills, not procrastinating, and spreading out study time to avoid stress. Students recommend attending all classes because this may be the only time (due to the lack of time) that you can see the material.

The faculty are described as caring, conscientious, and demanding, with high expectations of student performance. There are abundant opportunities for research with faculty; however, most students feel that there is little time for this during the regular school year. The placement rate is very good as a result of UCLA's excellent reputation. However, because the grading system is Pass/Nonpass, instructor recommendations, as well as National Board scores, are of great importance. Strong departments at UCLA dental school are Endodontics, Restorative Dentistry, and Pedodontics.

FINANCIAL

The cost of attending UCLA dental school for residents, who make up the vast majority of the class, is relatively inexpensive, with the exception of housing. Students figure the total cost for the first year from $7000 (resident living at home) to approximately $14,000 for nonresidents. Obviously, the cost of living in the area around the school is a major factor in this figure. Students buy their instruments for about $5000 with payment primarily over the first two years.

SOCIAL LIFE

Students find that there are definitely opportunities for social interaction, particularly in the first year. Social events such as TGIF parties and alumni day are sponsored by the dental school, and several social events are put on by the undergraduate campus. The students describe themselves as relaxed and mature individuals who "Don't get stressed out for every test." They are friendly, social, helpful, and caring. This school attracts an outstanding group of dental students who are willing to "go that extra mile."

COMMENTS: It is hard to beat UCLA for a quality dental education. The faculty are very good, the school is moderately priced (relative to other dental schools) for in-state residents, and it is among the top dental schools in the nation. The students work very hard but feel the grading system allows them a chance to absorb more information under less pressure.

UNIVERSITY OF CALIFORNIA/SAN FRANCISCO
School of Dentistry
San Francisco, California 94143

LOCATION: Big City

AGE OF SCHOOL: 107 Years

CONTROL: Public/State

AADSAS **MEMBER:** Yes

CLASS SIZE: 88

PERCENT WOMEN IN CLASS: 39

PERCENT MINORITIES IN CLASS: 47

AVERAGE STUDENT EXPENDITURE: $ (In-state); $$ (Nonresident)

POSTDOCTORAL PROGRAMS: Yes—dental public health, orthodontics, pedodontics, periodontics, prosthodontics, oral and maxillofacial surgery, and general practice residencies

PHYSICAL ENVIRONMENT

University of California/San Francisco School of Dentistry is very beautiful, with a spectacular view of San Francisco and the bay area. The school, an attractive building surrounded by greenery, was built in 1980 and is accessible to other facilities, including the Milberry Gymnasium, which has a pool, weights, racquetball courts, and Ping-Pong tables. A new library, described by one student as "extra beautiful and big," will be completed in 1990. The medical library is easily accessible, as is the Berkeley Campus, which is across the bay. The clinics are very new and well kept, particularly the sophomore clinic, which is the biggest and is very modern. The dental clinic is in excellent condition.

The area around the school has had some safety problems in the past. It is difficult to find housing near the dental school, and an average one-bedroom apartment near the school averages $450 per month. Apartments are the most common form of housing. Students feel that having a car would definitely be beneficial, but it is not absolutely necessary because public transportation is available.

ACADEMICS

Students recommend taking histology and physiology along with art classes (including sculpting) before entering dental school. Tests are graded fairly most of the time and competition for good grades is present. Morphology lab is the hardest course because it requires great skill and understanding together with high teacher expectations. It is considered the best course at the dental school. Keeping up with lecture material and reviewing works well for students at this school. Students spend about four hours a night studying. The faculty are outstanding in their field of research; many are world-renowned as well as very friendly. Opinions are mixed about the faculty's teaching abilities, but all students agree that the level of instruction received, along with recent research, is outstanding. Orthodontics, Pedodontics, and Oral Surgery are considered to be among the strongest departments.

FINANCIAL

Because the school is state supported, UC/San Francisco costs less than many other dental schools. The total cost of the first year of dental school costs an in-state student about $14,000, and a nonresident about $16,000. Students purchase their instruments for approximately $6500, with payment primarily during the first two years. There is not much time for work outside of school.

SOCIAL LIFE

UC/San Francisco dental school affords its students limited opportunity to socialize outside of class due to commitments to studies. In addition, there are few students outside of the health sciences schools. Other students find that the mixture of students from other health schools is very stimulating. The school attempts to encourage socializing by planning such activities as dances, movies, parties, and picnics. The class is outgoing, although groups of students tend to "stick together."

COMMENTS: As one of the best dental schools in the nation (particularly clinically), UC/San Francisco attracts a highly motivated student body with diverse interests. Most students here are from California. The quality of instruction is slightly uneven; however, students find their overall education more than justifies the school's outstanding reputation. A very enthusiastic student sums up her first thoughts at UC/San Francisco: "The knowledge here is never-ending. It is stressed here that the mere acquistion of facts does not suffice; it is the importance of wisdom that is most appreciated."

UNIVERSITY OF COLORADO
School of Dentistry
4200 E. Ninth Avenue / Denver, Colorado 80262

LOCATION: Urban/Big City

AGE OF SCHOOL: 21 Years

CONTROL: Public/State

AADSAS MEMBER: Yes

CLASS SIZE: 35

PERCENT WOMEN IN CLASS: 40

PERCENT MINORITIES IN CLASS: 15

AVERAGE STUDENT EXPENDITURE: $ (In-state); $$$ (Nonresident)

POSTDOCTORAL PROGRAMS: No

PHYSICAL ENVIRONMENT

The University of Colorado School of Dentistry is housed in a new, modern building located near Colorado General Hospital. There is no planned renovation of the clinical or basic sciences facilities, but students say, "There is no need [to renovate]. We have very modern equipment." The clinic is very well run and highly efficient. The school borders both low and middle income housing areas and the area around the school is considered fairly safe if proper precautions are exercised at night, including traveling in pairs and "not taking risks."

There are no gym facilities at this school; however, discount memberships are available at several local athletic clubs. Students will find a number of restaurants, theaters, and shopping areas within easy access of their school. It is advised that if possible, students bring a car to get around Denver. It is not difficult to find both suitable and affordable housing near the school, although most of it is rather old and lacks some modern conveniences. The average cost for a one-bedroom apartment in the area of the school ranges from $275 to $350 per month.

ACADEMICS

Students at this school take primarily basic sciences the first two years and clinical courses the remaining two years. Student exposure to patients generally occurs during the third year. A new General Practice Internship/Externship Program provides students with a chance to practice dentistry in a variety of settings during the last year, including geriatric centers, hospitals, public clinics, and child care centers. These extramural experiences are mixed with intramural rotations where the student learns about the dental speciality of his or her interest. Students attend school through the summer.

The small class size at Colorado enhances the educational experience for students because they find that they have more interaction with clinical professors. It is not the material itself that makes the classes difficult but rather the volume. Students recommend taking art classes—sculpting, painting—and biochemistry, along with any classes that you "really wanted to take." Grades are based on a numerical system translated into letters of A(90–100), B(80–89), C(70–79), and D(60–65). Students find that the classes are not competitive and "everyone works to help one another." Biochemistry, pharmacology, and gross anatomy are among the hardest basic sciences at this school. It is recommended that students be very organized, take notes on all required readings, and attempt to prepare themselves so that they don't need to cram for exams.

There are many opportunities for research, which students can conduct during elective time during their last two years. Students have a very good opinion of the faculty at this school. They say that the faculty really care about student performance and making certain that students understand the material rather than memorize it.

FINANCIAL

The first year at Colorado School of Dentistry will cost the average in-state student about $17,000, and nonresidents about $27,000. Students buy their instruments for a total of about $6000, with payment primarily during the first two years thus making the third and fourth year considerably less expensive. Most students take out some form of federal loans and the school offers limited aid to students who demonstrate extreme financial need.

SOCIAL LIFE

There are numerous activities planned for students. The small class size gives the school a "family" type of feeling. Students here are not cutthroat and are willing to help one another during tests. There are a good number of nonresidents and some older students in the classes.

COMMENTS: Colorado's small class size provides the distinct advantage of good opportunities for individual attention, which is important in any dental school. The faculty is considered good and the facilities are fine.

UNIVERSITY OF CONNECTICUT
School of Dental Medicine
263 Farmington Avenue / Farmington, Connecticut 06032

LOCATION: Rural/Small City

AGE OF SCHOOL: 20 Years

CONTROL: Public/State

AADSAS **MEMBER:** Yes

CLASS SIZE: 40

PERCENT WOMEN IN CLASS: 37

PERCENT MINORITIES IN CLASS: N/A

AVERAGE STUDENT EXPENDITURE: $ (In-state); $$ (Nonresident)

POSTDOCTORAL PROGRAMS: Yes—available in several dental specialities; also D.M.D.-Ph.D. program available for students interested in dental research and/or academic dental medicine

---

PHYSICAL ENVIRONMENT

University of Connecticut School of Dental Medicine is housed with the medical school in one very large, very modern, and very interesting looking white building. The school itself is surrounded by Farmington, a quaint New England town that is beautiful in the fall and has many outdoor activities, such as skiing, close by. The area around the school is relatively safe, and most students have not heard of any problems with security. The facilities in the dental school clinic are excellent. Although the fourth-year lab area is crowded, the other three years' labs are very spacious. Overall, students are very pleased with the facilities present in their dental school.

Housing is a major source of concern and complaint among students. Though there are no dorms for dental students, it is relatively simple to locate housing near the dental school. Unfortunately, much of this housing is inordinately expensive. One-bedroom apartments near the school cost $650 per month. Some students suggest obtaining less expensive housing by traveling 10 miles from the school. The Health Science Center is 40 miles from the main campus, so the students compensate for not having main campus facilities by going to nearby gyms. The student government gets students discounts at two YMCAs and at a Jewish Community Center. Transportation other than walking is necessary, and for that reason, most recommend having a car.

ACADEMICS

The courses vary greatly in their level of difficulty, but most students agree that it's the sheer volume of work that weighs them down. The university's Committee System is such that students often take only one or two courses at a time. As one woman puts it, "You just immerse yourself!" Students at this school recommend taking mammalian life sciences. "Take mammalian biology courses. Not plants or fungi—mammals." They also feel that art classes, such as drawing or sculpting, would be good preparatory courses because of the development of manual dexterity. Other suggestions include taking biochemistry and having a familiarity with histology.

The university's School of Dental Medicine is a rarity among most dental schools in that the courses are Pass/Fail. Students should be forewarned that the method of determining what is a "Pass" is based on class performance. Needless to say, competition for grades is not totally alleviated. After all, nobody wants to be under the cutoff for "Pass." Students here take their classes with the medical school for the first two years; there is not much difference between the curricula, with the exception of some additional dental classes. Cellular and molecular biology, anatomy, and central nervous system are among the hardest courses. Students feel that keeping up with work instead of cramming (which is often tempting) is the way to succeed.

The faculty are regarded highly, and because of the small class size, individual attention is afforded to students. There are numerous research opportunities, including summer research fellowships that offer stipends of approximately $1600. Periodontics, Restorative Dentistry, and Oral Surgery are considered strong departments.

FINANCIAL

University of Connecticut is a fantastic buy as far as dental education goes. In-staters pay about $12,000 per year, while their out-of state counterparts pay $17,000. Students purchase some of their instruments. Jobs are available through the school. One student works in a hospital as a lab technician, but she says that it is not easy to work because of the demanding schedule. Loans are a must for most students, and the university has a very good financial aid office for those in need of help.

SOCIAL LIFE

Contrary to the myths, the School of Dental Medicine is not entirely made up of Connecticut residents. It is harder for out-of-staters to get accepted to the school, but there are students from other states here. The school makes a special effort to ease the transition for first-year students by providing advocacy groups for first- and second-year students. There are many social functions, such as a film series, parties, coffee houses, and the Gong Show which is a lighthearted look at the faculty. The students are from diverse backgrounds and strive to become topnotch dentists.

COMMENTS: University of Connecticut School of Dental Medicine provides students with a reasonably priced dental education. The school maintains high standards and will cut its class size before admitting students with mediocre or poor scholastic credentials. This not only ensures that the students admitted are of high caliber, but also maintains the very good reputation of this school.

UNIVERSITY OF DETROIT
School of Dentistry
2985 East Jefferson / Detroit, Michigan 48207

LOCATION: Urban/Big City

AGE OF SCHOOL: 56 Years

CONTROL: Private (Religious affiliation: Catholic)/State Support

AADSAS **MEMBER:** Yes

CLASS SIZE: 62

PERCENT WOMEN IN CLASS: 30

PERCENT MINORITIES IN CLASS: 10

AVERAGE STUDENT EXPENDITURE: $ (Both in-state and nonresident)

POSTDOCTORAL PROGRAMS: Yes—offered in conjunction with numerous dental specialties

---

PHYSICAL ENVIRONMENT

The facilities at the University of Detroit School of Dentistry are a combination of both old and new. The school is made up of four buildings that are located away from the undergraduate campus. There is a modern classroom building that houses faculty offices, an anatomy lab, and a student lounge. The clinic is an older four-story building that is currently undergoing renovation. All dental equipment is "state of the art." The dental library is an interesting feature of the school because it is a restored 19th-century home.

Obtaining suitable housing can be difficult since the housing surrounding the school is "project and low-income housing." It is not advised to seek housing in this neighborhood, and most students rent and share houses in the surrounding suburbs, which they say are "very good deals." A one-bedroom apartment costs between $200 and $250 per month. A 15- to 45-minute drive is considered average to get to the school from these suburbs. The area surrounding the school is not particularly safe, but one student counters that "the area of the school is perceived as much worse than it actually is and there is adequate protection at the school."

ACADEMICS

The courses are considered far more advanced and in-depth as compared to undergraduate courses. Some students remark that the courses are "geared towards dentistry," so the courses are more challenging since the material is very new to them. Competition for grades seems present, but students are willing to help each other out. Along this line, one student suggests that studying with a partner is an effective method but make sure that it is not a "teacher-student" relationship, but rather a partnership with someone who is academically equal to you.

The students have suggested taking Latin, medical terminology, biochemistry, histology, physiology, and a basic business management course before entering. Anatomy and pharmacology are among the hardest courses for students. Prosthetics, Oral Surgery, and Endodontics are considered strong departments. Students do not find that they have much problem locating patients. There is a definite clinical emphasis at this school, which students enjoy a great deal.

FINANCIAL

Students expect the first year of Detroit School of Dentistry to cost about $15,000 next year. Students buy their instruments, as well as articulators, for approximately $6500, with payment due primarily over the first two years of study. Most students take out GSL, HPL, and Perkins Loans. HEAL loans are used only as a last resort. It is possible to work during your time at Detroit, and the school attempts to set up work/study jobs. However, if at all possible, it is best not to work because of the amount of schoolwork.

SOCIAL LIFE

There are many social events planned for students at Detroit dental school including an open house, the Belle Isle Bash, ASDA Day, and the ASDA Dance. Students at this school are hardworking, responsible, and outgoing. This school offers students outstanding clinical experience. As one student sums it up, "Being a small, private school, the students and faculty put in a serious effort to work together and make things run as smoothly as possible."

COMMENTS: The facilities are fine and the cost of attending this school is reasonable for in-staters. Although the location is not among the best, the school has maintained an excellent reputation as a quality dental school.

UNIVERSITY OF FLORIDA
College of Dentistry
Box J-445 / Gainesville, Florida 32610

LOCATION: Suburban/Medium Sized City

AGE OF SCHOOL: 16 Years

AADSAS **MEMBER:** Yes

CLASS SIZE: 77

PERCENT WOMEN IN CLASS: 23

PERCENT MINORITIES IN CLASS: 21

AVERAGE STUDENT EXPENDITURE: $ (In-state); $$(Nonresident)

POSTDOCTORAL PROGRAMS: Yes—available in conjunction with numerous dental specialties

---

PHYSICAL ENVIRONMENT

The University of Florida College of Dentistry is located within the University of Florida health science center. The building is 10 years old and made of red brick. Renovation of the inside is expected to be finished in 1989. As one student remarks, "This brick building with the little trees is my home." There are three floors of student clinics for patient care.

The dental school facilities are only a few blocks from university facilities, and there is a good bus system that picks up students outside of the school. There are several shopping malls, movies, and cultural events. The dental school is in a suburban and relatively safe area.

Finding housing is "A piece of cake . . . with lots of cakes to choose from." The school is located in a big suburban area with a lot of available housing. The cost for furnished single apartments ranges from $220 to $500 per month. Dorm rooms are available for about $1500 a year.

ACADEMICS

Students feel that their courses are far more extensive than what they encountered as undergraduates. However, because of the way the material is organized, it is fairly easy to learn. Students recommend courses that help develop manual dexterity, such as sculpting or painting, as well as biochemistry, behavioral psychology, and microbiology. The curriculum eases students into clinical work and also gives them a degree of freedom with numerous elective courses.

Many students at the College of Dentistry are interested in post-graduate training. Among this group the competition for good grades is intense. Neuroscience and immunology are among the hardest basic sciences courses encountered by students. Endodontics, Oral Medicine, and Operative Dentistry are considered to be very strong departments.

The faculty are excellent and get along well with students. There are opportunities for student research in every department. Students selected the school for its reputation, cost, faculty, and facilities.

FINANCIAL

University of Florida College of Dentistry runs about $12,000 for a single in-state resident and approximately $17,000 for nonresidents. Many (in-state) students here do not consider loans a must but feel that they are an enormous help. GSLs as well as school loans are recommended. It is possible to buy used equipment and apply for scholarships in order to reduce costs. Instruments are generally bought for a total of $6500, with the bulk of the cost occurring during the first year. The school provides limited working opportunities and discourages students from having "regular" jobs due to the time restraints imposed by the schoolwork. However, there is enough time to work if a student must to afford the school. Paid research positions are available.

SOCIAL LIFE

Although there are many social events at this school, students feel that it undeservedly gained a reputation as a "party school," which it certainly is not. The dental fraternities here are very active socially and there are parties before football games, picnics, and intramural activities.

COMMENTS: The University of Florida College of Dentistry offers students a fine dental education with an emphasis on clinical training. The class is warm, friendly, well-rounded, hardworking, and very satisfied at having chosen this school.

UNIVERSITY OF IOWA
College of Dentistry
Iowa City, Iowa 52242

LOCATION: Small City

AGE OF SCHOOL: 106 Years

CONTROL: Public/State

AADSAS **MEMBER:** Yes

CLASS SIZE: 72

PERCENT WOMEN IN CLASS: 13

PERCENT MINORITIES IN CLASS: 7

AVERAGE STUDENT EXPENDITURE: $ (Both in-state and nonresident)

POSTDOCTORAL PROGRAMS: Yes—M.S. programs in conjunction with community dentistry, fixed and removable prosthodontics, endodontics, operative dentistry, oral pathology/diagnosis, oral and maxillofacial surgery, pediatric dentistry, and periodontics

PHYSICAL ENVIRONMENT

The University of Iowa College of Dentistry is housed in a fairly new building, approximately 15 years old, which has very modern laboratory and clinical facilities. As a result of the school's proximity to the main campus, there are ample athletic facilities for students to use. A new cafeteria is currently being built on the lower floor of the dental school building.

The area surrounding the school is considered fairly safe and one student describes it: "It has all the advantages of most major cities with the security and friendliness of a smaller town." It is not difficult to find housing near the school, and the cost for a two-bedroom apartment (per person) is between $250 and $300 per month plus utilities. Most students at the dental school choose to live in apartments. It is recommended that students bring a car, but most feel that it is not absolutely necessary.

ACADEMICS

The courses are much more demanding than those in undergraduate school. Students recommend taking histology, business, accounting, computers, finance, and courses fostering manual dexterity before entering. They feel that it is unnecessary to take upper-level chemistry courses because you will not require them once here. Competition for good grades, particularly A's, is intense, but it is less intense for B's and C's. Students found pharmacology, histology, systemic disease manifestations, and gross anatomy to be among the hardest courses at the school.

It is recommended that students keep up with their reading assignments, study with a partner, and use mnemonics. The professors are considered good, and most are genuinely interested in the students. There are several opportunities for student research, as well as special-care programs in which students work with the medically compromised, the elderly, and veterans. Students have their first exposure to patients during the first year. Operative Dentistry, Prosthetics, and Oral Surgery are considered very strong departments here; however, this is also an excellent school for general dentistry.

FINANCIAL

The cost of attending Iowa is about $10,000 for the average in-state student and approximately $15,000 for nonresidents. Students buy their instruments over the first three years of school for approximately $5000. Many students take out GSLs, and the school does award some scholarships to students with excellent academic records. There are some part-time jobs offered by the school, but students feel that first-year students should not work because of the extreme limitations on their time.

SOCIAL LIFE

Students find plenty of time at Iowa College of Dentistry to attend dances, gatherings organized by social clubs, and the dental school's formal dinner dance. Most students are from Iowa, and there are a sizeable number of women preparing for a second career in the class.

COMMENTS: This school attracts a highly capable and interesting student body. The facilities are more than adequate, and there are excellent opportunities for extramural clinical experience.

UNIVERSITY OF KENTUCKY
College of Dentistry
Lexington, Kentucky 40536

LOCATION: Suburban

AGE OF SCHOOL: 26 Years

CONTROL: Public/State

AADSAS **MEMBER:** Yes

CLASS SIZE: 40

PERCENT WOMEN IN CLASS: 25

PERCENT MINORITIES IN CLASS: N/A

AVERAGE STUDENT EXPENDITURE: $ (In-state and nonresidents)

POSTDOCTORAL PROGRAMS: Yes—available in conjunction with numerous dental specialties; also, combined B.S.-D.M.D. program with the University of Kentucky

PHYSICAL ENVIRONMENT

The University of Kentucky College of Dentistry buildings are fairly new. Students feel some renovation could be done, but they add that any needed equipment is always provided to the student. The dental school is near campus and athletic facilities, with the Seaton Sports Center right next to the Medical Center. A gym is located across the street, and there is a campus bus service that runs every 15 minutes to get you anywhere you wish to go on campus.

Students are in love with the area surrounding their school. The location is a medium-sized city near the most beautiful thoroughbred horse farms in the country. The area around the school is very safe.

It is not hard to find housing in Lexington, which has many apartments, houses, and duplexes for rent or sale. The cost of housing is reasonable, with a one-bedroom apartment ranging from $250 to $280 per month and a two-bedroom costing about $340 per month. Apartments are the most common form of housing.

ACADEMICS

It is necessary to be more organized than as an undergraduate because you take so many courses at the same time. The difficulty of courses ranges from easier than college to much harder. Students encourage predents to take courses that teach them how to "deal with people," such as public speaking or psychology. Also recommended are biochemistry, histology, and independent research, if possible.

Tests are graded fairly, and competition for good grades is intense because of increased competition for GPRs (general practice residencies) as well as specialty programs. The hardest courses are neuroanatomy, facial pain, head and neck, and histology. Flash cards as well as "excellent notes" are advised for students wishing to do well in courses at Kentucky College of Dentistry. The faculty are very interested in both the students and research and have an excellent relationship with most students. Oral Pathology, Restorative Dentistry, and Oral Diagnosis are considered very strong departments.

FINANCIAL

Students buy their articulator and handpiece at Kentucky dental school for approximately $3700, with most of the payment due over the first two years. They rent their other instruments for about $2200, payment for which is spaced out over the four years. The school year is about $10,000 for residents and $15,000 for nonresidents. Loans are available from both the university and the dental school. Most students have loans. They do not recommend working during the first year.

SOCIAL LIFE

Kentucky dental students are very "close and social." There are several social events, many of which are sponsored by the ASDA, including a Halloween Party, the ASDA Banquet, and other parties.

COMMENTS: Kentucky gives preference to in-state applicants, but some out-of-staters are accepted each year. This school has a very good tutorial program, and both administrators and faculty work to help students whenever problems are brought to their attention. Students at this school are bright and highly motivated.

UNIVERSITY OF MARYLAND
College of Dental Surgery
666 West Baltimore Street   /   Baltimore, Maryland 21201

LOCATION: Big City

AGE OF SCHOOL: 148 Years

CONTROL: Public/State

AADSAS **MEMBER:** Yes

CLASS SIZE: 96

PERCENT CLASS WOMEN: 30

PERCENT CLASS MINORITY: 25

AVERAGE STUDENT EXPENDITURE: $ (In-state); $$ (Nonresident)

POSTDOCTORAL PROGRAMS: Yes—available in conjunction with numerous dental specialties; also, combined B.S.-D.D.S. programs with several colleges, including University of Maryland/College Park, University of Maryland/Baltimore, Bowie State College, Coppin State College, and Morgan State University

---

PHYSICAL ENVIRONMENT

University of Maryland College of Dental Surgery is in a relatively new building within a small graduate campus made up of a variety of both old and new buildings. Students feel that the school is centrally located but lacks nonacademic facilities. The gym is at the top of a parking garage, and there are no athletic fields for student use. The facilities within the dental school are nice and comfortable. The clinical area is scheduled for a complete renovation in the next two to three years. The clinic will be equipped to use light-operated handpieces in the near future.

The area surrounding the school is a paradox. To the west and north the area has low-income housing; to the south and east it is a glitzy, fashionable, expensive area—all within eight blocks of the school. Housing is not difficult to find and costs about $350 per month for a one-bedroom apartment in the area of the school. Apartments and shared houses are the most common form of housing. For the most part, the area around the school is relatively safe if students exercise a degree of caution when they walk about at night.

ACADEMICS

Students feel it is the time consumed by classes that makes the courses difficult at Maryland. However, one student says, "If you have the discipline to study when you get home, you will be an 'A' or 'B' student." Predents planning to go here are advised to take psychology courses as well as computer software, economics, and business management. Pharmacology is among the most challenging courses because it involves a lot of memorization and takes a great deal of time. "You cannot study it in one or two nights. You must understand physiology to help." Long hours, good notes, and continuous studying are recommended for doing well here. Periodontics, Fixed and Removable Prosthodontics are all considered very strong departments at Maryland School of Dental Surgery.

The faculty are considered very accessible and most are also "very good conveyers of information and lab techniques." There are several opportunities for student research, as well as a closed-circuit television center and photographic and art studios. Students do not find that there is a great deal of competition for grades.

FINANCIAL

Students buy their instruments at Maryland. In-state students spend on the average $12,000 for the first year; nonresidents pay about $16,000. Grants are available for state residents, which decrease costs considerably. Maryland does have a work/study program, but students do not recommend working, especially in the first year.

SOCIAL LIFE

There are a variety of social events for students at Maryland School of Dental Surgery, including Skit Nite, dances, trips, and a charity ball. Students here are well mixed. They are very positive about their school because they are aware of the high caliber of students in their classes as well as of Maryland's reputation for turning out quality dentists.

COMMENTS: There are several nonresidents admitted to this school, although it is more difficult for them to get in than it is for in-staters. Maryland is a top notch school of dentistry by any standard, with ample opportunities for interaction with faculty and for student research.

UNIVERSITY OF MICHIGAN
School of Dentistry
Ann Arbor, Michigan 48109-1078

LOCATION: Suburban/Medium-Sized City

AGE OF SCHOOL: 113 Years

CONTROL: Public/State

AADSAS **MEMBER:** Yes

CLASS SIZE: 100

PERCENT WOMEN IN CLASS: 30

PERCENT MINORITIES IN CLASS: 15

AVERAGE STUDENT EXPENDITURE: $ (In-state); $$ (Nonresident)

POSTDOCTORAL PROGRAMS: Yes—M.S. and Ph.D. programs available in conjuction with numerous dental specialties

---

PHYSICAL ENVIRONMENT

University of Michigan School of Dentistry is in a modern, well-maintained structure located one block from the main campus and houses a Dental Research Institute. The school is situated in a relatively safe and suburban area. There are exceptional sports facilities near the dental school, including the central campus recreational building. The business and entertainment districts of Ann Arbor are close by as well.

The dental clinics are easily accessible and the cubicles are set up in the clinic for maximum convenience. Some equipment is beginning to show wear from age, but most is still good. There is a large, comfortable waiting room for patients. The lecture halls are in good condition and have modern video-audio equipment.

It is not difficult to find suitable housing in the area of the dental school, but what is around is not cheap. An unfurnished apartment near the school ranges from $490 to $550 per month. Apartments are the most common form of housing used by the students.

ACADEMICS

One student says "Getting an 'A' in certain courses is like winning the state lotto and just as easy!" On a more serious note, students recommend that predents take physiology, interpersonal communications, some advanced psychology, and as many basic sciences as possible. Pharmacology and gross anatomy are considered the hardest courses because of the amount of material, and operative clinic and lectures are difficult because of the grading, which, as stated earlier, makes it difficult to achieve an 'A'. A nice feature of the school's curriculum is that the dental faculty teach applied oral science courses in conjunction with basic sciences courses in order to relate what the students are learning in their medical school classes to dentistry.

Students stress group studying for gross anatomy, which helps you get to know other students as well as "bounce information off of each other." The vast majority of the faculty are very enthusiastic and progressive. Operative Dentistry, Oral Diagnosis, and Oral Pathology are considered to be very strong because the instructors are excellent. Students selected Michigan based on its outstanding reputation as well as its cost.

FINANCIAL

Michigan School of Dentistry will cost about $15,00 for residents and $20,000 for nonresidents the first year. Students currently buy their instruments at the school for a total cost of approximately $6000, with the majority of payments occurring over the first two years. It is possible to work after the first year and during summers. Many students take advantage of National Student Direct Loans (NDSL) as well as grants and scholarships offered by the school.

SOCIAL LIFE

There are many social activities planned for dental students, including parties, recreational sports, raft trips, Practice Management Day, and the Christmas party. The majority of the class is easygoing and relaxed, but students still work hard and help one another in lab or clinic if needed.

COMMENTS: Michigan has the advantage of an outstanding national reputation coupled with a very reasonable cost for in-state students. The school has excellent faculty, research opportunities, and clinical facilities.

UNIVERSITY OF MINNESOTA
School of Dentistry

15-106 Malcolm Moos Health Sciences Tower
515 Delaware Street, S.E. / Minneapolis, Minnesota 55455

LOCATION: Urban/Big City

AGE OF SCHOOL: 100 Years

CONTROL: Public/State

AADSAS **MEMBER:** Yes

SIZE OF CLASS: 104

PERCENT WOMEN IN CLASS: 36

PERCENT MINORITIES IN CLASS: 3

AVERAGE STUDENT EXPENDITURE: $ (In-state); $$ (Nonresident)

POSTDOCTORAL PROGRAMS: Yes—dental public health, endodontics, oral pathology, oral surgery, orthodontics, pediatric dentistry, periodontics, and prosthodontics

PHYSICAL ENVIRONMENT

The University of Minnesota School of Dentistry is located in the health sciences complex, which is made up of fairly new buildings. The school is within two blocks of the main campus and one block of the student union and gym. There are numerous restaurants and bars across the street. Safety is not thought to be a major problem, although it is advised that students walk in groups at night.

Students consider the dental school's facilities to be excellent and "state of the art." The school's central sterilizing unit is among the best in the country. The school is located about a mile from downtown Minneapolis. Housing is not difficult to find, although it may be harder to locate *both* a worthwhile and affordable place to live. Much of the housing around the area of the school is expensive, with a one-bedroom apartment averaging $350 to $450 per month. Most students choose to share houses.

ACADEMICS

Minnesota integrates basic sciences with clinical material both during and after each course. Students find their faculty to be "excellent teachers who want you to know the latest advances in dentistry up to the minute." During the second year students begin their formal treatment of patients. There are also electives offered during this year, but the majority of electives occur during the fourth year. Numerous extramural opportunities exist for students, including clinical work at geriatric facilities, a free clinic in St. Paul, and several hospital sites, such as the VA, St. Paul Ramsey Hospital, and Hennepin County Medical Center. Opportunities for research are available especially during the summer session.

Competition for grades is not intense, but some "gunners" are present in the classes. Biochemistry, humanities, and art courses are recommended before attending this school. Students find biochemistry to be among the most challenging of the basic sciences. There are many learning aids, including computer instruction, slides, and television movies. Taking good notes, attending all lectures, and studying in groups are methods students suggest for academic success at this school.

FINANCIAL

The total cost will be approximately $12,000 for first-year in-state students and $17,000 for nonresidents. Most students take out a loan of some sort, and the school is reputed to have a fine financial aid office. Students pay a fee of about $700 each year for using their instruments, which is a major cost savings over purchasing instruments. It is not recommended that students work their first year, but after that it is considered possible and the school finds jobs for students.

SOCIAL LIFE

Minnesota students find that they have time for a social life after they are finished attending classes, doing lab work, and studying for exams. There are parties sponsored both by the school and students, but as one student mentions, "The attendance could be better." A significant number of nonresidents attend the school, and the class as a whole is diverse, highly motivated, and caring.

COMMENTS: The faculty and facilities are the strongest features at this school. Minnesota offers its students a solid preparation for a career in dentistry and numerous extramural opportunities, including several area hospitals and other facilities.

UNIVERSITY OF MISSISSIPPI
School of Dentistry
2500 N. State Street   /   Jackson, Mississippi 39216-4505

LOCATION: Suburban/Big City

AGE OF SCHOOL: 15 Years

CONTROL: Public/State

AADSAS MEMBER: Yes

CLASS SIZE: 35

PERCENT WOMEN IN CLASS: 10

PERCENT MINORITIES IN CLASS: 5

AVERAGE STUDENT EXPENDITURE: $ (In-state); $$ (Nonresident)

POSTDOCTORAL PROGRAMS: No

PHYSICAL ENVIRONMENT

The University of Mississippi's School of Dentistry is one of the newest buildings at the Mississippi Medical Center (UMMC). The buildings associated with the dental school are very modern. Although there is no gym on the UMMC campus, there are a basketball court and an intramural football field on the campus. There are health clubs and a YMCA available for a nominal fee.

Mississippi dental school is in a safe area about two or three miles from downtown Jackson. UMMC provides limited on-campus housing for students on a first-come, first-served basis. There are plenty of apartments within driving distance of the dental school. Two-bedroom apartments range from $350 to $400 per month, while one-bedroom apartments range from $250 to $340 per month. Apartments are the most common form of housing used by students. Mississippi dental school's clinical facilities are modern.

ACADEMICS

Students at Mississippi dental school are enthusiastic about their system of being grouped into teams with a student from each class, from freshman year. The senior student presents the case, and the professor asks questions of the "team." This gives students early exposure to patients as well as a chance to ask questions from more experienced students. Dental students begin to treat their own patients at the end of the second year. Unlike many dental schools, Mississippi dental school does not take its basic sciences classes with the medical school. Students like this because more time is devoted to "dental-related knowledge."

Biochemistry, business management, and psychology are recommended courses for prospective students. Biochemistry, material science, and pharmacology are considered among the most difficult courses encountered by students at Mississippi dental school. Daily studying is the easiest method for doing well in courses at this school. Endodontics and Fixed Prosthodontics are considered strong departments at this school.

FINANCIAL

Students at Mississippi do not buy their instruments. They rent them for a cost of about $2300, payable in four equal installments over the four years of study. Depending on residency the cost of attending for the first year ranges from $7000/ (resident) to $15,000/ (nonresident). Cost also depends a great deal on living accommodations and your personal style of living. Loans are considered a "must" here, and students say that it is possible to work during junior and senior years. The school also provides job opportunities for students.

SOCIAL LIFE

There are several social events at Mississippi dental school, including golf tournaments, many parties, and Christmas and Spring balls. Sudents are very diversified at this school as well as personable, bright, and concerned.

COMMENTS: Mississippi combines the best approaches to dental education by providing its students with early exposure to patients yet, at the same time, allowing them to "ease into the process" by working with older, more experienced students. The school's facilities are very good and modern, and there are numerous opportunities for student research. This is an excellent dental school for any predents to consider, particularly Mississippi residents.

UNIVERSITY OF MISSOURI/KANSAS CITY
School of Dentistry
650 East 25 Street   /   Kansas City, Missouri 64108

LOCATION: Big City

AGE OF SCHOOL: 25 Years

CONTROL: Public/State

AADSAS **MEMBER:**   Yes

CLASS SIZE: 120

PERCENT WOMEN IN CLASS: 23

PERCENT MINORITIES IN CLASS: 18

AVERAGE STUDENT EXPENDITURE: $ (Both In-state and nonresident)

POSTDOCTORAL PROGRAMS: Yes—available in conjunction with numerous dental specialties

PHYSICAL ENVIRONMENT

The dental school is housed in a blonde brick building with aqua trim. The school is about three miles north of the main campus. The "Hospital Hill Gym," located about two blocks from the school, has weights and a basketball hoop. However, one student who uses the gym laments that it is overrun with nursing students doing aerobics.

The dental school facilities are more than adequate, and the clinic has just acquired new A-Dec equipment and chairs. Planned renovation includes a new denture lab, waiting room, and offices. The school is next to the Crown Center, Truman Medical Center, Children's Mercy Hospital, the Pershing Memorial, and the Hyatt Regency.

The school is situated in a neighborhood of mostly low to lower middle SES, so students can find housing easily. There are no dorm rooms, but housing near the school is not very expensive. A one-bedroom apartment runs about $200 per month. There are several forms of housing including apartments, sharing houses, and renting rooms.

ACADEMICS

The work is slightly less difficult than undergraduate work. The difficulty arises from poorly worded exams, redundant questions, and typos on written tests, as well as from heavy lab courses with numerous deadlines. Students say "Contrary to what undergraduate advisors recommend, forget diversity or novelty in selecting courses. It is important to have a solid background in human anatomy, physiology, microbiology, and biochemistry." Competition here is very intense for good grades. Students are very concerned with being accepted into specialty programs and general practice residencies.

People who can easily memorize notes and textbooks will have a decided advantage at this school. However, simply memorizing material will probably result in a mediocre grade, so students must understand what they're reading as well. The introduction of a new dean has changed the traditionally clinical outlook, which has dramatically shifted toward being one that is research-oriented. Many students feel that this change has happened too quickly. Although the end results of this will benefit newer students, upperclassmen have become embittered over this sudden movement.

Opportunities for research here are excellent. It has even been suggested that research may soon become a requirement (in some form) to graduate. Students selected this school for its outstanding clinical reputation. Although they are disgruntled over the changes taking place several students still believe their clinical instruction is adequate. Among the strongest departments are Pediatric Dentistry, Operative Dentistry, and Endodontics.

FINANCIAL

Students buy their instruments for about $3000 the first year and $1600 the second. The cost of the first year for a single student runs approximately $12,000 for residents and $15,000 for nonresidents, including tuition, books, living expenses, and materials. The university has a tuition agreement with Arkansas, Kansas, and New Mexico. Students in these states pay in-state tuition at the dental school. It is possible to work. A few jobs are provided by the school, but the pay is not considered very good.

SOCIAL LIFE

There are many social opportunities for students outside the classroom, such as professional groups (ASDA, ASDC), women's groups (AAWD), and spouse support groups. There are also class parties, all-school parties, and educational meetings. Most students here are serious and mature.

COMMENTS: The student situation at this school is difficult at present, but many students believe that "things will improve in the coming years, hopefully sooner." You should be aware of the shift presently going on from a clinical to a heavier research orientation.

UNIVERSITY OF NEBRASKA—LINCOLN
College of Dentistry
40th and Holdrege / Lincoln, Nebraska 68583-0740

LOCATION: Suburban/Small City
AGE OF SCHOOL: 71 Years
CONTROL: Public/ State
AADSAS **MEMBER:** Yes
CLASS SIZE: 56

PERCENT WOMEN IN CLASS: 20

PERCENT MINORITIES IN CLASS: N/A

AVERAGE STUDENT EXPENDITURE: $ (In-state); $$ (Nonresident)

POSTDOCTORAL PROGRAMS: Yes—endodontics, orthodontics, pedodontics, periodontics, and oral and maxillofacial surgery; also, M.S. and Ph.D. programs available in conjunction with oral biology

PHYSICAL ENVIRONMENT

The Lincoln College of Dentistry is nicely landscaped. Its location next to an arboretum gives it a peaceful setting. The building was built in 1967, but the facilities are kept up to date and are very well maintained. The school is on the east campus of the University of Nebraska, which is somewhat removed from the main campus. There are several lighted tennis courts and outdoor basketball courts just behind the dental college. The school is only a short walk from the new east campus student center and a small gym.

There has been a slow upgrading of the operative chairs, and the student lounge areas have been renovated. Students find that the school takes great pride in fixing any dental equipment that breaks down. The area surrounding the school is considered relatively safe.

One student describes Lincoln as "a city that has a big town appearance but the atmosphere of a small town." It is not difficult to find reasonably priced housing in the area of the school. A one-bedroom apartment (furnished) costs approximately $260 per month. Apartments are the most popular student housing. Students recommend bringing a car if possible.

ACADEMICS

The courses here are far more difficult than undergraduate courses. However, one student adds a comforting comment: "But [the courses are] not so hard that they can't all be completed." Students recommend taking biochemistry ("a must") and business courses, as well as having a familiarity with anatomy. According to one student, "The UNMC freshman anatomy course weeds out the weak." "Gunners" are not altogether uncommon, and most students agree that competition for good grades is intense here.

Anatomy ("the professor is fantastic and demands a lot from his students"), pathology, and operative technology are considered among the hardest courses encountered by students. It is suggested that very accurate note-taking is necessary for good performance on exams, as well as reviewing every night after the lectures.

The student/faculty relationship at this school is very good. Most of the professors/doctors will go out of their way to help a student. There are many opportunities for student research, but because of the demands of the first year, it is not advised to conduct research during freshman year. Restorative Dentistry and Endondontics are considered strong departments at this school.

FINANCIAL

The average in-state student will spend about $14,000 for the first year. Nonresidents will pay about $18,000 for their first year. After living in Nebraska for six months, students can qualify for in-state tuition. Students pay a total clinical fee of about $10,000 spread out in equal payments over the four years. Most students take out GSLs and find there is not much need to take out many other forms of loans. There does not appear to be a problem with working—even several freshmen have jobs—but it is suggested that you refrain from working the first year if at all possible. There are also some summer research jobs provided by the school.

SOCIAL LIFE

There are many social activities at the College of Dentistry, including a golf tournament in the fall known as the Molar Open, a pig roast put on by the junior class, a casino raffle in the spring sponsored by freshmen, a freshman-sophomore picnic, Spring Day, and a Halloween Party.

COMMENTS: This dental school has an outstanding and highly competitive student body, good faculty, and very adequate facilities. Extramural clinical experiences are readibly available to students in a variety of settings, including hospitals and private dentists' offices.

UNIVERSITY OF NORTH CAROLINA
School of Dentistry
Chapel Hill, North Carolina 27514

LOCATION: College Town

AGE OF SCHOOL: 38 Years

CONTROL: Public/State

AADSAS **MEMBER:** Yes

CLASS SIZE: 75

PERCENT WOMEN IN CLASS: 35

PERCENT MINORITIES IN CLASS: 5

AVERAGE STUDENT EXPENDITURE: $ (In-state); $$ (Nonresident)

POSTDOCTORAL PROGRAMS: Yes—available in conjunction with numerous dental specialties; also, D.D.S.-Ph.D. program in conjunction with basic sciences and D.D.S.-Masters of Public Health (M.P.H.) available.

PHYSICAL ENVIRONMENT

Many students feel that UNC stands for the University of Neverending Construction. The University of North Carolina dental school is no exception to this, for it is always being remodelled and updated. However, this is done in such a way as to not inconvenience students. The dental school is a relatively new building attached to an old one. The interior is always clean and is nicely decorated. The most modern equipment is in dental education and research.

The laboratories, clinics, and facilities are of the latest technology. Planned renovations are in progress to provide more clinical space. There are also plans to computerize student-patient clinic schedules.

The university has an efficient and convenient shuttle-bus system. Main campus facilities are within a 5- to 10-minute walk. The gym is also very close to the school. Parking seems to be the major problem for students and faculty.

Chapel Hill is 25 miles from Raleigh, the state capital, and 10 miles from Duke University. The city is in the middle of a housing boom. One year ago it was more difficult to find housing than it is today. However, housing and living costs are the highest in the state.

Apartments range from $400 to $900 per month. Most students prefer this type of living accommodation.

ACADEMICS

Students would definitely recommend that prospective students take anatomy or at least have a familiarity with the subject before entering the dental school. They also suggest taking a course to improve reading speed and comprehension. Tests are graded fairly, and competition is very much present until after the first semester, when "things quiet down." Microbiology, pathology, and gross anatomy are among the most difficult courses encountered. Study methods include team studying as well as reviewing every night and on weekends.

Student/faculty ratios are low at the university. Faculty are genuinely interested in students. There are vast opportunities for research, especially since UNC's Dental Research Center is among the top-ranking centers in the country. Career counseling is strong here, with lectures given by experts in practice management, attorneys, and accountants.

FINANCIAL

Regardless of state residency, UNC is a bargain for the quality of education offered. Students buy their instruments during the first two years for about $5000 (divided up). The cost for a first-year in-state student is about $15,000. Out-of-state students pay approximately $20,000 for the first year. Many students attempt to change their residency in order to reduce the cost of tuition. Loans are the norm for most students, especially to cover the cost of buying instruments. It is not possible to work during the first year; after that it is easier because there are fewer time-consuming, didactic classes. The school has an excellent work/study program.

SOCIAL LIFE

There are many social activities at the dental school. There are dental fraternity parties, the annual schoolwide picnic, and class parties. The students have diverse backgrounds.

COMMENTS: UNC School of Dentistry is a first rate dental school with an interesting and highly motivated student body. Those who choose this school will not be disappointed. The clinical and research facilities, faculty, and cost of attending this school are very good. There are a considerable number of out-of-state students (about 15 percent) admitted to the class.

UNIVERSITY OF PENNSYLVANIA
School of Dental Medicine
4001 Spruce Street   /   Philadelphia, Pennsylvania 19174

LOCATION: Urban/Big City

AGE OF SCHOOL: 110 Years

CONTROL: Private

AADSAS **MEMBER:** Yes

CLASS SIZE: 75

PERCENT WOMEN IN CLASS: 25

PERCENT MINORITIES IN CLASS: 10

AVERAGE STUDENT EXPENDITURE: $$$$ (Both In-state and nonresident)

POSTDOCTORAL PROGRAMS: Yes—available in conjunction with numerous dental specialties; several combined programs including D.M.D.-Master Business Administration (M.B.A.) available through the Wharton school as well as D.M.D.-M.D; also, biodental 6-year program through University of Pennsylvania/College of Arts & Sciences undergraduate, 6-year program through Rensselaer Polytechnic Institute, 7-year program through Lehigh University; Bryn Mawr College also has a combined program with the dental school

PHYSICAL ENVIRONMENT

The University of Pennsylvania (Penn) dental school is an older, Ivy League–looking building situated on the university campus. The school is at the farthest corner of the campus, making on-campus facilities quite a walk while off-campus facilities are next door. The area around the school is relatively safe, although women would be advised to walk in groups at night. The dental school is a beautiful facility with up-to-date equipment and immaculate operatories. First-year students take most of their classes in "the dungeon," the basement of the school, which has no windows.

Finding housing at Penn is not difficult. The average cost for a one-bedroom apartment is from $350 to $400 per month. Although there is a student dormitory, off-campus housing is preferred by most students. Having a car is not really necessary because of the good mass-transit (bus) system around the school.

ACADEMICS

The material at Penn School of Dental Medicine is not more difficult, just greater in volume, than undergraduate material. Comparative anatomy, biochemistry, and histology are recommended before entering this school, as well as liberal arts courses. As one student puts it, "Enjoy all the liberal arts you can in undergrad. You won't see them here."

All dental classes are taught apart from medical classes. This provides students with more of a focus on "dental areas," such as intensive study of the head and neck in gross anatomy. Penn's philosophy, however, is that the patient is a person and not just a mouth, and so the school also emphasizes humanistic approaches to dentistry. Tests are computer graded and competition for good grades is relatively strong because of the letter grading system. (Pluses are used but not minuses). Students find anatomy to be one of the hardest courses. Daily studying is seen as the best way to do well in courses. The faculty here are mixed, with some being very enthusiastic about their course matter and students and others being interested only in their research. Strong departments are General Restorative Dentistry, Oral Surgery, and Endodontics.

There are more opportunities for student research than there are students to take advantage of these opportunities. The school itself has a strong philosophy that dentistry is a specialty of medicine and the dentist is treating a patient rather than an oral cavity.

FINANCIAL

Students buy their instruments. Many use their summer income from the year before they enter dental school to pay off part of these costs which is approximately $5000. There are different finance programs to pay for instruments, but one student suggests that it is much cheaper to pay for them straight out if possible. A year at Penn School of Dental Medicine is about $30,000 for a single student. Almost all students take out GSLs and NDSL loans; many also take out HEAL loans. The school provides some jobs for students, but it is not advised that first-year students work. Some students (especially in the second and third year) work in dentists' offices doing clerical and/or computer programming jobs. Students bemoan the high cost of attending Penn but offer this piece of advice, "You pay for what you get. You want to come out of one of the top dental schools in the country. It's not cheap."

SOCIAL LIFE

There are many social activities at Penn School of Dental Medicine. Many of these are organized by the three coed dental fraternities on campus. The school organizes parties, and the students have occasional "happy hours" as well. Students here are tightly knit, but there are a lot of strong personalities attracted to this school.

COMMENTS: Penn proved itself one of the wiser dental schools by cutting its class size in a time when applications to dental school were down. There are numerous crossover programs between the dental school and the Wharton School of Business, the law school, and medical schools (not Penn's). One student warns, "These look appealing, but by the time you're done paying for your dental education there isn't much left to pay for another school." Penn is definitely among the top dental schools in the country and continues to attract very bright, articulate, and highly capable dental students.

UNIVERSITY OF SOUTHERN CALIFORNIA
School of Dentistry
Room 124 University Park-MC0641 / Los Angeles, California 90089

LOCATION: Urban/Big City
AGE OF SCHOOL: 91 Years
CONTROL: Private
AADSAS **MEMBER:** Yes

SIZE OF CLASS: 120

PERCENT WOMEN IN CLASS: 25

PERCENT MINORITIES IN CLASS: 30

AVERAGE STUDENT EXPENDITURE: $$$$ (Both in-state and nonresident)

POSTDOCTORAL PROGRAMS: Yes—avaialable in conjunction with several dental specialities; M.S. and Ph.D. programs with craniofacial biology; also, the International Student Program for foreign dental school graduates

PHYSICAL ENVIRONMENT

The University of Southern California (USC) School of Dentistry is housed in the Norris Center. The school's facilities and clinic are outstanding and there are closed-circuit televisions in labs and classrooms for instruction. The school has its own production studio where it tapes instructional programs for its students to watch in the lab.

A major benefit at USC is the dental school's affiliation with numerous hospitals at which students are able to do extramural internships. Among these hospitals are the innovative facility Rancho Los Amigos Hospital, Los Angeles County/USC Medical Center, which has a good variety of patients, and Children's Hospital.

The area surrounding the dental school is considered fairly safe by students. USC is located within a short drive of athletic clubs, and there are athletic facilities on the undergraduate campus. It is not difficult to find suitable housing near the school. One-bedroom apartments range from $350 to $400 per month. Most students prefer this form of living accommodation. Students find that having a car is very helpful at this school.

ACADEMICS

USC teaches students using a diagonal curriculum whereby students start out taking mostly basics sciences and end up learning mostly in the clinic. Competition for good grades (letter grades are used) is rather high particularly among the top students in the class. It is recommended that predents take biochemistry and work with a dentist or a dental specialist to gain manual dexterity skills, which will come in handy in the lab.

Students praise the faculty for their outstanding lectures and presentations of original research. Says one student, "You've got some of the best dentists on the West Coast teaching here." Implantology is a course considered to be "on the cutting edge." Students recommend studying in small groups, taking good notes, and paying careful attention to lab techniques in class. There are numerous opportunities for student research, particularly during the fourth year, through both honors and special elective programs.

FINANCIAL

The first year is the toughest financially because students pay $5000 toward their instruments (a total of $8000) this year. The total cost of the first year for students is approximately $27,000. Almost all students take out a loan of some sort. The financial aid office is considered very helpful. Students feel that it is not feasible to work while enrolled at this school.

SOCIAL LIFE

USC attracts a number of nonresidents each year. The class is "friendly, outgoing, and very social." There are numerous student gatherings, as well as school-sponsored parties.

COMMENTS: USC School of Dentistry is an excellent school and has a fine location, excellent faculty, and very good clinical facilities, including even a mobile clinic. The cost for attending is rather high, but one student says, "You have to invest in order to profit and this place is a great investment."

UNIVERSITY OF TENNESSEE/MEMPHIS
College of Dentistry
875 Union Avenue / Memphis, Tennessee 38163

LOCATION: Big City
CONTROL: Public/State
AADSAS **MEMBER:** No

CLASS SIZE: 90

PERCENT WOMEN IN CLASS: 23

PERCENT MINORITIES IN CLASS: 10

AVERAGE STUDENT EXPENDITURE: $ (In-state); $$ (Nonresident)

POSTDOCTORAL PROGRAMS: Yes—orthodontics, oral surgery, pedodontics, periodontics, and general practice residencies

PHYSICAL ENVIRONMENT

The University of Tennessee (UT)/Memphis Dental School, the oldest state-supported dental school in the South, is made up of pleasant-looking modern buildings. There are an athletic field and a gym that are similar to those of a health spa, a student center, dorms, and parking lots close to the dental school. The school and clinic are both in excellent condition, and for the present time, there is no need for renovation.

The dental school area is safe during the day, but during the night it can be unsafe. Security guards will drive students to their cars at night. Most students feel that having a car is very important. It is difficult to find housing near the school. The cost for an average one-bedroom apartment is approximately $285 per month. Most students live in apartments.

ACADEMICS

Students recommend taking biochemistry before entering dental school, along with art and business classes. Tests are graded fairly, and competition for good grades (the school uses a letter system of grading) is present Very few students receive A's (an A is from 95 to 100%). Most grades resemble a bell curve with the majority of students getting B's and C's and very few failures. Pharmacology is the hardest course. Students strongly recommend studying old exams for all classes.

The faculty here are very fair-minded and attempt to help students whenever needed. Operative Dentistry, Crown and Bridge, and Oral Pathology are considered very strong departments. Abundant research opportunities exist for students. Most students selected the school for its outstanding clinical facilities.

FINANCIAL

The total cost to attend UT/Memphis for in-state students is about $15,000 for the first year. Nonresidents pay about $3000 more per year. It is not easy for out-of-staters to transfer residency once they begin attending the school. Students buy their instruments for approximately $7000, with the bulk of the payment due during the first and second years. Many share apartments and live-on campus in order to save money. Some students do work during the school year, but this is not advised by students.

SOCIAL LIFE

There are many chances for socializing outside of the classroom setting at the dental school. Fraternity parties, class parties, and campus events afford students the chance to break away from their books, especially on weekends. Students here are easy going and attempt to help each other.

COMMENTS: The UT/Memphis College of Dentistry has excellent clinical facilities, a fairly good location, and a very reasonable cost for both in-staters and nonresidents. The school offers numerous opportunities for research, and the students have a very positive outlook about their school.

UNIVERSITY OF TEXAS
HEALTH CENTER AT SAN ANTONIO
Dental School
7703 Floyd Curl Drive / San Antonio, Texas 78284

LOCATION: Outskirts Big City

AGE OF SCHOOL: 18 Years

CONTROL: Public/State

AADSAS **MEMBER:** No

CLASS SIZE: 100

PERCENT WOMEN IN CLASS: 21

PERCENT MINORITIES IN CLASS: 15

AVERAGE STUDENT EXPENDITURE: $ (In-state); $$ (Nonresident)

POSTDOCTORAL PROGRAMS: Yes—prosthodontics, periodontics, endodontics, pediatric dentistry, general practice residencies, and oral surgery residency; also, D.D.S.-M.S. and D.D.S.-Ph.D. programs available

PHYSICAL ENVIRONMENT

The University of Texas Health Center at San Antonio (UTHCSA) Dental School is housed in a modern building that has, students say, "among the finest clinical facilities in the country." One student, however, muses that the patient waiting room "resembles a bus depot." Most students are very enthusiastic about the fact that they are assigned a cubicle during their first two years for studying and later, a fully equipped cubicle that simiulates a dental office.

UTHCSA Dental School is close to numerous athletic facilities, including a track, basketball courts, tennis courts, and volleyball courts. There is also easy access to nearby research hospitals. There are no dormitories for students, but it is not difficult to find reasonably priced housing, which averages $260 per month for a one-bedroom apartment. The school is located in a very large city that has many cultural opportunities and shopping areas (San Antonio is the tenth-largest city in the U.S.) and is considered relatively safe. Mass transit is available, but students find that having a car is a "major plus."

ACADEMICS

Students strongly recommend taking Spanish, comparative anatomy, physiology, and art courses before attending this dental school. There is some competition for grades (a letter system). One student feels that "getting A's is very difficult but after that it's not so bad." Students have their first patient experience during the first year ("very minimal"), and by the fourth year, they are in the clinic most of the time.

The faculty at this school are considered very caring and highly informative. Students comment that there are several retired military people on the faculty ("They use to call our school Wilford Hall East after the air force base across town") who are "rigorous" with material, but all faculty go out of their way to make certain their students receive extra help when they need it.

It is recommended that students study old exams, and many students here advocate "cram sessions." Gross anatomy and physiology are considered among the hardest basic sciences. Operative Dentistry, Crown and Bridge, and Orthodontics are considered very strong departments.

FINANCIAL

Tuition at this school is graduated, with a continual increase throughout the four years. The first year will cost a total of $10,000 for residents and $17,000 for nonresidents. Students buy their instruments for approximately $7500, with the majority of payment over the first two years. Most students take out some sort of loan, and the school awards limited funds to students who demonstrate financial need. It is not recommended that students work while enrolled at this school because of the limitations on their time.

SOCIAL LIFE

Students at this school boast that there is a very good social life here. There are many social activities, including Friday happy hours in the cafeteria, Fiesta de Tejas once a year, the annual dental school olympics, and several keg parties. Students are from a broad spectrum of backgrounds, and there is a significant number of nonresidents in the classes.

COMMENTS: Students here believe that you can have fun at the same time you are attending dental school. The faculty are good, and the clinical facilities are outstanding. This school should be considered by anyone interested in a topnotch dental education in an area with a warm climate.

UNIVERSITY OF WASHINGTON
School of Dentistry
D323 Health Sciences Building / Seattle, Washington 98195

LOCATION: Medium-Sized City
AGE OF SCHOOL: 43 Years
CONTROL: Public/State

AADSAS **MEMBER:**   Yes

CLASS SIZE: 50

PERCENT WOMEN IN CLASS: 24

PERCENT MINORITIES IN CLASS: 28

AVERAGE STUDENT EXPENDITURE: $ (In-state); $$ (nonresident)

POSTDOCTORAL PROGRAMS: Yes—endodontics, fixed prosthodontics, oral medicine, orthodontics, periodontics, and removable prosthodontics: also: M.S. and Ph.D. programs available in conjunction with oral biology

PHYSICAL ENVIRONMENT

The University of Washington's dental building is one large wing of the immense Health Sciences complex overlooking Portage Bay Yacht Basin on Lake Union. The clinics are clean, well-equipped, and spacious. Most of the facilities in the dental school are up to date, and the building has been adapted to meet the needs of modern dental equipment. However, students do have to keep their equipment in pushcarts.

The Health Sciences center is only about a 5- to 10-minute walk from the campus sports complex. The university is 20 minutes from downtown Seattle, and there are many shopping and entertainment facilities nearby for students. Housing is not difficult to locate if students get an early enough start (about a month before starting classes). The average one-bedroom apartment costs between $300 and $350 per month. Most students live in apartments.

ACADEMICS

The volume of material is very heavy at University of Washington, but students do not find the courses conceptually more difficult than their undergraduate science courses. Students recommend that predents take biochemistry, physiology, histology, developmental biology, and psychology. Competition is not as high as has been rumored at this school, and students sincerely attempt to help one another when tests are near. Gross anatomy and pathology are among the hardest basic sciences for students.

Group study appears to be a successful study method. One student adds, "Constant quizzing in these groups pounds the information into your brain." Most important is to read the syllabus, because the classes are based more on these than on texts. The professors are considered very good educators and willing to help students who need it. There are ample research opportunities offered by the school.

FINANCIAL

The average in-state student will spend a total of about $13,000 ($20,000 for nonresidents) for the first year. Students buy their instruments for approximately $7800, with the majority of payment occurring over the first and second year of study. Most students take out a combination of loans, and there are some grants offered by the school. It is not recommended that students work because of the severe time limitations.

SOCIAL LIFE

There are opportuities for social interaction at this school ranging from student-faculty get-togethers to class-organized parties. Students tend to break off into groups. There are a significant number of nonresidents and some older students.

COMMENTS: This school has the benefits of a first-rate faculty, great facilities, a nice location, and a very reasonable cost for residents. There are some very good extramural clinical opportunities for seniors. As far as the students are concerned, the rumors about the classes being cutthroat are generally unfounded.

VIRGINIA COMMONWEALTH UNIVERSITY
Medical College of Virginia School of Dentistry
Box 566   /   Richmond, Virginia 23298

LOCATION: Urban/Big City

AGE OF SCHOOL: 95 Years

CONTROL: Public/State

AADSAS **MEMBER:** Yes

CLASS SIZE: 90

PERCENT WOMEN IN CLASS: 10

PERCENT MINORITIES IN CLASS: 15

AVERAGE STUDENT EXPENDITURE: $ (In-state); $$ (Nonresident)

POSTDOCTORAL PROGRAMS: Yes—oral surgery, orthodontics, endodontics, periodontics, oral pathology, pediatric dentistry, fixed and maxillofacial prosthodontics, and dental anesthesia

PHYSICAL ENVIRONMENT

Virginia Commonwealth University (VCU) School of Dentistry is made up of two interconnected buildings. The school is housed within the Medical College of Virginia (MCV), which has a gym, hospital, and dining and student center all within easy access of the dental school. Although VCU School of Dentistry is nearly 100 years old, the facilities are in very good condition, and a fiber optic system is currently being installed for use with handpieces.

The school and its surrounding area do not appear to be unsafe. Also, a downtown renovation project in the area of the school appears to be quite successful. Many students choose to live in on-campus housing, which is considered adequate for student needs. The majority of students find housing in nice, quiet areas about 20 minutes from the campus. The cost of housing varies a great deal, with a room in a three-person apartment costing between $150 and $200 per month plus utilities. Students suggest bringing a car to school if possible.

ACADEMICS

Students find that courses at this school are more difficult in theory and especially in quantity of work than undergraduate course work. Very few A's are awarded to students, but the level of competition for grades is relatively low. There is "far more of a common spirit or goal" than in college. Physiology, dental anatomy (because the graded projects are quite difficult), and complete dentures are among the hardest courses.

The faculty are considered excellent and are "genuinely interested in student concerns." Students believe that the large number of full-time faculty is a large factor in the high quality of instruction they receive. There are several research opportunities, but they are limited to summer programs. It is recommended that prospective students take biochemistry, histology, business courses, and art and sculpture prior to entering dental school. Oral Surgery, Endodontics, Periodontics, and Crown and Bridge are considered very strong departments by students.

FINANCIAL

The cost of attending the School of Dentistry for in-staters is about $14,000 for the first year. Nonresidents will spend approximately $19,000 for their first year. Students purchase their instruments for approximately $5000, with payment primarily during the first two years of school. Most students take out loans in the form of GSLs, and the school grants several scholarships, many of which are exclusively for the first year of study. Approximately 30 percent of the class are employed part-time in such areas as the dental clinic in the hospital.

SOCIAL LIFE

There are many opportunities for social interaction at the dental school because MCV is located within its own campus. There are private parties or school-sponsored events almost every weekend. The dental school also has its own guest speakers and social events. Although students in the dental school are individuals with diverse interests, the class is closely knit. As one man sums it up, "We are dedicated yet very 'laid-back.' "

COMMENTS: This school offers outstanding social science courses in practice management and professional ethics. The students here are enthusiastic about both the faculty and the administration. VCU provides its students with a solid foundation in dentistry and a full array of postdoctoral programs that enrich their understanding of dental specialties.

THE
MEDICAL
SCHOOLS

ALBANY MEDICAL COLLEGE
47 New Scotland Avenue   /   Albany, New York 12208

LOCATION: Urban/Medium-Sized City

AGE OF SCHOOL: 149 Years

CONTROL: Private

AMCAS **MEMBER:** No

CLASS SIZE: 150

PERCENT WOMEN IN CLASS: 30

PERCENT MINORITIES IN CLASS: 5

AVERAGE STUDENT EXPENDITURE: $$$ (In-state and nonresident)

M.D.-Ph.D.: Yes—biochemistry, microbiology-immunlology, pathology, and physiology;

BIOMEDICAL PROGRAMS: Accelerated—6-year program with Rensselaer Polytechnic Institute and 7-year program with Union College; nonaccelerated—8-year program with Siena College

NBME **Part I:** Students must take and record a score.

NBME **Part II:** Students must take and record a score.

PHYSICAL ENVIRONMENT

Some call it the "Little City," but most Albany students are more than satisfied with the location of their school. Albany Medical College is situated near downtown Albany, along with the Albany Medical Center Hospital Complex. Although there is no college campus around the school (Union College, which the school is affiliated with, is half an hour away), there are many facilities built within the school. There are a student lounge, weight-lifting center, bookstore, coffee shop, and two gyms in the buildings adjacent to the medical center. The safety of Albany Med's location is a drawing point for many students applying to the school. There are several hospital sites. The most widely used among these facilities is Albany Medical Center Hospital (AMCH), which is also considered the most efficient facility. Medical students have access to modern labs and computer facilities, including the planned installation of LION (Library Information Online Network), a computerized listing of all the books from Albany Med, the Capital District Psychiatric Center, and the Albany College of Pharmacy. The VA hospital is across the street, and although it is not talked about in glowing terms, there is a renewed interest in the hospital because students feel they are given more hands-on opportunities with patients there. St. Peter's is a "low-key" hospital that Albany students like a great deal. They are paged as "Dr." on the intercom and are generally treated very well by the staff. Ellis Hospital is in Schenectady, which is a 25-minute drive from Albany Medical Center Hospital, and offers the advantage of seeing a broad base of patients from every socio-economic group because it is the only hospital serving over twenty counties. The school's trauma center is currently being expanded. The Capital District Psychiatric Center is a large, well-run facility that is a neighbor of the school.

Some students wish they could have more patient involvement than they do in their first two years. However, third- and fourth-year students say that the last two years more than compensate for the heavy academics of the first two years. Students speak highly of the faculty and their instructors' receptiveness to meeting on an individual basis with students who have questions or need help.

Many students live in the dorm shared with Albany Law School their first year and choose to live in shared houses their next three years. Housing is not difficult to find and costs vary from $150 per month for a one-bedroom apartment to $500 to $600 per month for a three-bedroom rental.

The medical school's facilities are fairly new. There is a lot of renovation going on, including the completion of new labs. Lockers are available for students, although there are no private study carrels except in the library. Although Albany Med has no campus, there are many offerings in the Albany area, including the South Mall downtown, Saratoga Perfoming Arts Center, several area shopping centers, and more than a few adequate nightclubs.

ACADEMICS

Students feel that the heavy work load and not the work itself is what makes the courses at Albany Med so much more difficult than undergraduate courses. Recommendations to premeds for courses besides the required premed courses included biochemistry ("A must!"), literature, art, philosophy, and music or anything that has nothing to do with science, because there is enough science to be studied once there. One student felt that speed reading would be a handy course because of the volume of material to be read.

The great majority of students feel that tests are graded fairly. Although most students feel that competition for grades is not intense (Albany uses a modified Pass/Fail/Honors/High Honors system), rivalry for top grades is definitely present. Students have several choices for the "most difficult" classes—physiology, microbiology, pathology, and anatomy, which is only a semester compared to two semesters spent on pathology. Both pathology and anatomy are involved courses, with pathology putting emphasis on "little facts" and anatomy having a greater volume of material to master. There are numerous elective courses offered at the school, including computers in medicine, geriatrics, biomedical engineering, and medical jurisprudence.

Albany Medical College students recommended a variety of study methods for doing well in the basic sciences courses—systematic studying, organized note-taking, and continuous review of material. The student-run note service is reputed to be very helpful when studying for major exams. The most important idea is not to fall behind on your work, because catching up is very difficult. Students who encounter special difficulties during the year, such as illness, are given the opportunity to be on a modified schedule that allows them more time.

The clinical faculty at Albany Med is described as being very strong. Although the basic sciences professors are a bit weaker, they are very accessible for questions about the material covered in lecture. There are definitely opportunities for student research, during both the school year and summer, which are particularly good in neuroscience, physiology, and pharmacology. Students spend a variable amount of time studying, averaging 4 to 6 hours a day in the first two years and 1 to 3 hours a day in the last two two years.

FINANCIAL

The cost for the first year at this school will be about $24,000. Albany Med has school-sponsored loan programs and a work/study program for those with financial need. Although there are work opportunities for students in the library or in the lab, it is not recommended because of the time consumed by the heavy work load. Most students at Albany Medical College are either utilizing loans (HEAL loans are very popular) or are enrolled in the Armed Services which pays their way in return for serving in the military.

SOCIAL LIFE

Students have several opportunities for social interaction. Every other Friday night a "Beer Blast" is held by the second-year medical class. There are day trips on weekends and occasional parties held by the faculty/administration as well as picnics, semiformals, and student-sponsored parties. The student body is diversified, with some older students, some married students, and younger biomedical students. The annual commencement celebrations take many students away from their books. All in all, students appear to be very tightly knit within their classes and help students from other classes as well.

Albany Med students are above all happy with the school they are attending. In the words of one woman, "My time at Albany Med has been fantastic. I have learned more about helping people than I ever thought possible."

COMMENTS: Albany Medical College offers students the opportunity to treat patients from a wide spectrum of backgrounds, while at the same time it is located in a more relaxed environment than a larger city, such as New York or Boston. The construction of the new trauma center, as well as other proposed renovations, adds to the already strong appeal of this medical school.

ALBERT EINSTEIN
College of Medicine
Yeshiva University
1300 Morris Park Avenue   /   Bronx, New York 10461

LOCATION: Suburban/Big City

AGE OF SCHOOL: 33 Years

CONTROL: Private

AMCAS **MEMBER:** Yes

SIZE OF CLASS: 170

PERCENT WOMEN IN CLASS: 40

PERCENT MINORITIES IN CLASS: 10

AVERAGE STUDENT EXPENDITURE: $$$ (Both in-state and nonresident)

M.D.-Ph.D.: Yes—Einstein Medical Scientist Training Program (MSTP) with opportunities for advanced work in biochemistry, cell biology, molecular biology, developmental biology, genetics, microbiology and immunology, pathology, pharmacology, physiology, biophysics, neuropathology, neuropharmacology, neurophysiology, and behavioral science; also, postgraduate programs through Sue Golding Graduate Division of Medical Sciences and Belfer Institute for Advanced Biomedical Studies.

NBME **Part I:** Optional

NBME **Part II:** Optional

PHYSICAL ENVIRONMENT

A larger-than-life-sized bust of Albert Einstein sits on top of a pedestal, overlooking the school that bears his name, amidst trees and several medical students relaxing before their day begins. Albert Einstein College of Medicine, an affiliate of Yeshiva University, is located in the northeast part of the Bronx. The Belfer Educational Center has topnotch basic sciences classrooms and laboratory facilities, as well as the Anatomy Museum, Pathology Museum, and a Self-Instruction Center. Library facilities at this school are also very good, with computerized databases such as MEDLINE and TOXLINE.

The athletic center, which is open and easily accessible for students, includes a swimming pool, basketball and racquetball courts, exercise and weight-training rooms, and even a suspended jogging track. Students find that they are able to "get away" to Manhattan, Long Island, and Westchester on the weekends.

Einstein is known for its outstanding clinical facilities. Bronx Municipal Hospital Center (BMHC) is one of the primary clinical sites for medical students. The facility houses a wide spectrum of SES patients and cases. The BMHC has a phenomenal burn center that maintains a skin bank for grafting as well as a very well-staffed and well-administered trauma center. Chanin Institute for Cancer Research is a very large facility staffed with some of the leading experts on cancer in the United States. The Montefiore Medical Center is an older facility made up of two acute-care hospitals. North Central Bronx Hospital, which is under the aegis of Montefiore, is a municipal hospital with outstanding and very modern facilities.

Albert Einstein College of Medicine is located in what students consider a realtively safe area. Locating both adequate and affordable housing near the school can be a problem for students who do not live in school-owned housing. The Low Residence Complex is considered "liveable." The apartments are air conditioned and cost about $260 per month for a studio, $370 per month for a one-bedroom apartment and $470 per month for a two-bedroom apartment. Students strongly recommend sharing apartments to cut down on living expenses. Rhinelander is another Einstein-owned housing complex for students that is close to the main campus. A two-bedroom apartment costs about $390 per month at this facility.

ACADEMICS

Although the first year consists primarily of basic sciences, there are several courses which introduce students to the clinical aspects of medicine. Students are very enthusiastic about the course entitled Human Behavior and Psychiatry for the Physician, which is taught using small discussion groups under the tutelage of social workers, psychiatrists, and internists. During the first year students also have electives whereby they observe and participate in a chosen clinical program for between 13 and 20 consecutive Mondays. Students begin their formal clinical training during the second semester of the second year.

Competition among students for grades (Honors/Pass/Fail) is not only minimal but strongly discouraged at this school. Students recommend group studying, organized systems of studying such as outlining and note cards, and mnemonics. Students strongly recommend taking courses in both biochemistry and genetics because it is possible to place out of these courses through exemption exams. The faculty are spoken about in glowing terms. One student says, "They are so caring and easy to get hold of, that it almost makes you forget they're also so brilliant." There are outstanding opportunities for student research, ranging from M.D.-Ph.D. programs to independent study.

Another interesting opportunity for students exists through the Scientific Computing Center whereby qualified students can take courses in computer programming and learn the applications of statistical packages to biostatistics and areas of medicine. There are several international programs that are particularly strong between this country and Israel, including the Sharre Zedek Medical Center in Jersualem, through Hadassah, and the Shalom-Hartman Institute in Jerusalem. Other medical exchange programs also exist between Beijing, Paris, and Hanover, West Germany.

FINANCIAL

Einstein will cost the average single student approximately $25,000 for the first year of study. Most students take out some form of financial aid. According to most students, the financial aid office is highly receptive to students' financial needs, and some school scholarships and loans are available. It is not recommended that students work during the school year, but it is possible during summers.

SOCIAL LIFE

Human Dimensions is an interesting approach to help incoming students with anxiety and adjustment to medical school. The program consists of small groups supervised by faculty. Other activities include the Albert Einstein Symphony Orchestra, a film series, discount tickets to baseball games, and religious groups. The students at this school have firm beliefs regarding medicine and life in general and they are not afraid to express them.

COMMENTS: Although Einstein is only a little over 30 years old, it has established itself as one of the leading medical schools in this country. The administration has attempted (and succeeded) to integrate both clinical and basic sciences, offer boundless opportunities for student research, and provide an environment complete with outstanding clinical facilities, conducive to learning through an active interchange of information between students and faculty. One can only assume that had he been alive today, Albert Einstein would have been very proud of the medical school named for him.

BAYLOR COLLEGE OF MEDICINE
One Baylor Plaza / Houston, Texas 77030

LOCATION: Urban/Big City

AGE OF SCHOOL: 88 Years

CONTROL: Private with state support

AMCAS **MEMBER:** No

CLASS SIZE: 170

PERCENT WOMEN IN CLASS: 30

PERCENT MINORITIES IN CLASS: 5

AVERAGE STUDENT EXPENDITURE: $ (In-state); $$ (Nonresident)

M.D.-Ph.D.: Yes—audiology, biochemistry, cell biology, experimental biology, immunology, microbiology, neuroscience, pharmacology, physiology, and virology

NBME **Part I:** Optional

NBME **Part II:** Optional

PHYSICAL ENVIRONMENT

It is definitely Texas-sized. Baylor College of Medicine is the largest medical center in the United States. It is on a campus with two medical schools, three nursing schools, a high school for health professions, and dental and pharmacy schools. It has a total of approximately 7000 patient beds in eight hospitals. At present, there is over a *billion* dollars worth of construction going on within the medical center, including Methodist Hospital's new annex and the construction of a new nutrition center. The school's physical plant is excellent, with almost all facilities (with the exclusion of Ben Taub General Hospital, which is currently being rebuilt and is estimated to be completed in 1989) being very modern. The classrooms are spacious and have very good audiovisual aids.

There is not a campus per se (although Rice University is a half mile away); rather the main buildings are situated in the center of the medical center. Students have a new, small gym which is connected to the main building and is open seven days a week from 9 A.M. to midnight, as well as an aerobics room, a weight room, a cardiovascular room with bikes, and rowing machines.

There is an abundance of clinical sites, including several public facilities (Ben Taub County Hospital and Trauma Center, Jefferson Davis County Hospital, and the VA) and many private sites (St. Luke's Episcopal, Texas Children's, and the Methodist Hospital). Almost all hospitals are within a five-minute walk of the medical center. The school is located in southwest Houston in a fairly safe area. Housing is not difficult to find because it is currently a buyer's market. Condominiums (located in a "mini-city" with free bus access to the medical center) and apartments are the most popular form of housing with the cost of a one-bedroom apartment near the school ranging from $250 to $300 per month.

ACADEMICS

Students strongly recommend that premeds take physiology, bio-chemistry (because you can place out of it), and Spanish. The curriculum is set up so that students take basic sciences their first year and a half and have clinical experience during the remaining two and a half years. The students are graded Honors/Pass/Marginal Pass/Fail. Competition for Honors is apparent but confined to a small group of students. Physiology and pharmacology are considered among the hardest basic sciences because of their duration (four to six months), and students felt physiology was taught in such as way as to make it difficult to follow.

Study methods recommended by students include working with friends in study groups, mnemonics, and cutting classes to study the official class notes or syllabus. The faculty is approachable, but one student suggests, "You do need to approach them first, not the other way around." The anatomy department is considered very strong. There are numerous opportunities for research at this school. One student selected Baylor based on its clinical instruction, which she nows feels is " . . . so good it's overwhelming at times," and the access to so many teaching hospitals.

FINANCIAL

Baylor College of Medicine will cost approximately $8000 for the first year for in-state students and $19,000 for nonresidents. Students take out a variety of loans (primarily GSL), and there are some scholarships awarded by the school. There are work opportunities, such as lab jobs in the hospital where students can make between $24 to $48 a night that students can take late in their second year of study.

SOCIAL LIFE

There are several social activities for students, especially the first year, including the Annual Baylor Ball, Annual Senior Picnic, Annual Freshman Picnic, Senior Class Play, and Halloween parties. There are also intramural sports and special-interest clubs.

COMMENTS: As several students mention when talking about Baylor, it has the advantage of being a private school with state support, giving it the plus of having lower tuition for residents. The clinical facilities and research opportunities are extraordinary by any standard due to the size of the facilities (largest number of patients anywhere in the world) and the state-of-the-art clinical facilities that are currently expanding.

BOSTON UNIVERSITY
School of Medicine
80 East Concord Street / Boston, Massachusetts 02118

LOCATION: Urban/Big City

AGE OF SCHOOL: 140 Years

CONTROL: Private

AMCAS **MEMBER:** Yes

CLASS SIZE: 135

PERCENT WOMEN IN CLASS: 42

PERCENT MINORITIES IN CLASS: 15

AVERAGE STUDENT EXPENDITURE: $$$$ (Both in-state and nonresident)

M.D.-Ph.D.: Yes—available in conjunction with numerous academic areas; also, accelerated 6-year program available in conjunction with undergraduate program

NBME **Part I:** Optional

NBME **Part II:** Optional

PHYSICAL ENVIRONMENT

Construction is currently underway at University Hospital, amidst the older, more historic-looking buildings which together make up the Boston University Medical Center. The new addition at University Hospital, which will be completed by 1988, should alleviate some of the currently intense demand for both space and facilities. The basic sciences classrooms and laboratories are adequate for student needs. Clinical sites range from the very new to those needing repair. The hospital is in very good condition and has an excellent nursing staff and a wide variety of cases. The Boston City Hospital and the VA hospital are considered adequate teaching facilities.

Although the medical school is not located near the undergraduate campus, its facilities (which are rather extensive) are accessible by car. Boston University School of Medicine is located in a fairly safe area of Boston described as undergoing a "Yuppie gentrification," but caution is advised, especially at night. Housing around the school is expensive because Boston is currently a seller's market. Most students live in apartments, and students feel that it is difficult to find inexpensive housing that is both safe and close to the school. A one-bedroom apartment near the school costs between $550 and $600 per month.

ACADEMICS

Students find far less time to digest material than they had as undergraduates. It is recommended that prospective students take as many humanities courses as they can ("You'll get science for the rest of your life, but you won't get the liberal arts courses again") as well as biochemistry. Tests are graded fairly, and most professors will listen to comments about the tests. Competition among students is not intense because the medical school has an Honors/Pass/Fail grading system in which most of the class passes. There is no class rank, so most students compete against themselves rather than their classmates.

Pharmacology and pathology are considered among the hardest courses (they are taken at the same time) for students. In order to do well students should attempt to keep up with the work and make up review sheets to organize the material and study from later on. One student says, "Don't let it [the work] get to you (even if it feels like there's not enough time) . . . things will click."

The first and second years are all academic, whereas the last two years are primarily clinical. Students find that the faculty, particularly the clinical faculty, are responsive and very good teachers. There are numerous programs for research and several international programs, which students claim are among the most rewarding learning experiences of their medical education.

FINANCIAL

Boston University School of Medicine will cost the average student about $30,000 for the first year. Most students take out a combination of loans including GSL, HEAL, and Parent Loans (need-based,

$3000 per year up to a maximum of $15,000 with 12-percent interest and payment beginning 60 days after graduation). There are limited opportunities to work outside the classroom, including some lab jobs. However, students feel that the level of work prohibits having a job while enrolled at the school.

SOCIAL LIFE

There are opportunities for social interaction, but one student warns, "The student must take the initiative, because BU Med School is away from the main campus. The people one sees every day are fellow med students, not undergraduates or students in other graduate schools. . . . The opportunity to do extracurricular activities depends on the drive and organization of the individual." There are numerous parties at the school, including a fall and spring barbeque, a Christmas party, Skit Night, and a Match Day Party. Students have an active voice at this school and sit and vote on some of the faculty's standing committees. Numerous student organizations exist including the Primary Care Society; the Benjamin Waterhouse Society; Alpha Omega Alpha, an honorary fraternity; and Phi Delta Epsilon, a national medical fraternity.

COMMENTS: Students at this school mention that at times they feel overshadowed by the presence of Tufts and Harvard medical schools, but in all fairness, Boson University offers its students a very sound medical education and has an excellent track record of placing its graduates into top programs. The school's location is passable and the hospital sites are good. Perhaps the greatest strength of this school lies in its student body, which includes a diverse group of individuals ranging from accelerated biomedical students to members of the class who are in their late thirties and forties.

BOWMAN GRAY SCHOOL OF MEDICINE

Wake Forest University
300 South Hawthorne Road / Winston-Salem, North Carolina
27103

LOCATION: Suburban/Medium-Sized City

AGE OF SCHOOL: 47 Years

CONTROL: Private

AMCAS **MEMBER:**   Yes

SIZE OF CLASS: 108

PERCENT WOMEN IN CLASS: 33

PERCENT MINORITIES IN CLASS: 5

AVERAGE STUDENT EXPENDITURE: $$ (Both in-state and nonresident)

M.D.-Ph.D.:   No

NBME **Part I:**   Students must pass for promotion.

NBME **Part II:**   Students must pass to graduate.

PHYSICAL ENVIRONMENT

The Bowman Gray Medical Complex is a large conglomerate of modern buildings about a five-minute drive from the Wake Forest undergraduate (Reynolds) campus. Medical students have quick access to a track, playing fields, tennis courts, and the Winston-Salem YMCA. The school's basic science-laboratories and classrooms are in excellent condition. The library facilities are very good, with computer-assisted instruction (CAI) as well as access to MEDLINE and TOX-LINE, computerized bibliographies of the National Library of Medicine.

There are three main hospitals out of which students rotate. North Carolina Baptist Hospital, a well-staffed and efficiently run hospital next to the medical school, is the primary facility used by medical students. It houses intensive care, hemodialysis, rehabilitation facilities, and ambulatory care. Through the combination of Baptist with Forsyth Memorial Hosital, Reynolds Health Center (outpatient facility), and the Northwest Area Health Education Center, students are exposed to a very good variety of patients and cases.

Bowman Gray does not provide on-campus housing, but students say that it is not difficult to locate suitable accommodations, particularly with the help of the office of housing, which maintains a file of available rooms and apartments. The cost of a one-bedroom apartment near school is between $250 and $300 per month. The area around the school is considered safe. Students say that there is a definite problem with parking at this school.

ACADEMICS

This school introduced a new program for a small group of students in the fall of 1987. It is known as the Parallel Curriculum. This problem-based approach to medical instruction relies more heavily on independent instruction and self-directed learning. The students who volunteer and are selected for this program from those accepted at Bowman Gray are placed in groups of five to six students under the tutelage of a member of the faculty. The group uses selected cases to tie in both the basic and clinical sciences.

The remainder of the class is taught in the traditional methodology of basic sciences and clinical instruction. Students in this curriculum do not find that there is overt competition for grades (0.00 to 4.00 scale). They recommend taking biochemistry and social sciences such as psychology before entering. By and large, students find the faculty to be thoughtful, interesting, and innovative when attempting to explain difficult concepts. Research opportunities (some with a stipend) are available between school sessions. Students consider pathology and biochemistry to be among their hardest courses. It is recommended that students outline notes, attempt to get old tests, and study with a partner.

FINANCIAL

Bowman Gray will cost first-year students a total of about $20,000 regardless of residency. Students feel that having a job during the first year "may be detrimental to your health" due to the heavy work load that year. However, students do work, and the Office of Student Affairs will help students locate part-time employment. Most students take out some form of loan, and the school offers limited scholarships.

SOCIAL LIFE

Students at this school participate in a myriad of worthwhile organizations, including SOS (Students Offering Support). This group is run by students and involves medical students with activities at the Children's Home near the medical center. There are also several clubs, including the Student Medical Society, the Medical Student's Family Network, the Family Practice Club, the Student National Medical Association, AMSA, the American Medical Women's Association, The Gray Matter (student yearbook), On-Call (student newspaper), and the Christian Medical Society. The class is diverse, and students here are interested in both learning medicine and having meaningful interests outside the classroom.

COMMENTS: Bowman Gray offers several advantages to its students, including an outstanding faculty, good facilities and clinical sites, an enthusiastic and energetic student body, and a vital administration. The recent introduction of the Parallel Curriculum is a positive and progressive step in the enhancement of this fine medical school.

BROWN UNIVERSITY Program in Medicine
97 Waterman Street / Providence, Rhode Island 02912

LOCATION: Urban/Small City

AGE OF SCHOOL: 15 Years

CONTROL: Private

AMCAS **MEMBER:**   No

SIZE OF CLASS: 60

PERCENT WOMEN IN CLASS: 42

PERCENT MINORITIES IN CLASS: 15

AVERAGE STUDENT EXPENDITURE: $$$ (Both in-state and nonresident)

M.D.-Ph.D.:   Yes—biochemical pharmacology, biomedical engineering, ecology and evolutionary biology, molecular and cell biology, neurobiology and physiology

NBME **Part I:**   Passing score required for promotion

NBME **Part II:**   Passing score required for graduation

IMPORTANT: Since 1982 Brown has changed to a 7 to 8-year course of study. College juniors and seniors can gain admission to the school only through M.D.-Ph.D. programs and/or the Darthmouth-Brown Program.

PHYSICAL ENVIRONMENT

Brown University Program in Medicine is located in an attractive, modern facility that is integrated into the undergraduate campus.

The biomedical center is in very good condition, and the classrooms are very comfortable although they have no windows. The clinical sites are primarily older facilities that have been updated to keep pace with technological advancements. The Women's & Infant's Hospital was constructed a short time ago, and the Butler Hospital, a very well-run psychiatric center, is located on a nicely landscaped park. There are numerous conference rooms in the hospitals, and students find that there is ample study space.

Students have easy access to excellent athletic facilities on the main campus, including the gym, the ice hockey rink, the swimming center, and Nautilus equipment. Because the medical school is located on the main campus, students are able to take nonmedical school classes. The area around the school is considered safe, and students find no difficulty locating suitable housing, which averages between $250 and $300 per month for a one-bedroom apartment. Providence is centrally located, and many students travel to Boston on long weekends to "get away and forget the books."

ACADEMICS

Like Brown's innovative undergraduate education, the Brown Program in Medicine also offers a liberal approach to learning termed the Program in Liberal Medical Education (PLME). The majority of students are accepted to the medical school right out of high school and spend between 7 and 8 years at Brown. The goal of the program is for students to have an individualized education combining creative and original work with the study of basic and clinical sciences.

Competition for grades is not intense due in large part to the anonymous grading system that is used here. It is recommended that prospective students take biochemistry, genetics, embryology, statistics, and molecular biology in addition to several humanities courses and premedical requirements. Introduction to clinical training occurs in what are known as affinity groups. Affinity groups are designed to give students individualized attention while they learn such techniques as H&Ps (Histories & Physicals) and lab medicine.

The faculty are praised at this school for their compassion and understanding of the individual student's academic needs. There are outstanding opportunities for student research due to the "built-in freedom" inherent in the PLME. Students here do not recommend one set method for studying but do suggest that students be very self-motivated and disciplined in order to take advantage of as many educational opportunities as possible.

FINANCIAL

Brown will cost about $25,000 for both residents and nonresidents for the first year. Most students take out some form of loan. There are several job opportunities for those students who desire them, including lab jobs. Students recommend against working during the school year because of the time their studies take.

SOCIAL LIFE

Brown medical students have a unique opportunity for close interaction with undergraduate students. There are some social gatherings each year sponsored by the school and by groups of students. Most Brown medical students have known each other from the beginning of their undergraduate studies with the exception of students brought in from the M.D.-Ph.D. Program and students enrolled in the Brown-Dartmouth Program.

COMMENTS: This is one of the more interesting programs in medicine due to its inherent freedom. Brown is a school for the truly self-motivated individual who can use this freedom to its fullest and step outside the traditional sytem of medical education to enhance his or her understanding of medicine. The faculty, administration, and basic sciences facilities are all very good.

CASE WESTERN RESERVE UNIVERSITY
School of Medicine
2119 Abington Road / Cleveland, Ohio 44106

LOCATION: Urban/Big City
AGE OF SCHOOL: 145 Years
AMCAS **MEMBER:** Yes
CONTROL: Private
CLASS SIZE: 150
PERCENT WOMEN IN CLASS: 50
PERCENT MINORITIES IN CLASS: 10

AVERAGE STUDENT EXPENDITURE: $$$ (Both in-state and nonresident)

M.D.-Ph.D.: Yes—biochemistry, biomedical engineering, biophysics developmental genetics and engineering, molecular biology and microbiology, pathology, pharmacology, and physiology; also, separate M.D.-Ph.D. through Medical Scientist Training Program with anthropology, biology, biostatistics, epidemiology, macromolecular science, and reproductive biology

NBME **Part I:** Optional

NBME **Part II:** Passing score required for graduation

PHYSICAL ENVIRONMENT

Case Western Reserve University School of Medicine is located in a reasonably safe area. Students find the fact that the school is connected to the hospital by underground tunnels to be a big convenience during bad weather. The classes and labs (for first- and second-year students) have no windows, but they are all very comfortable and modern. The medical school is part of the main campus, and the gym is a three-minute walk away. A car is recommended for students to be "happy" and in order to get around, especially in the last two years.

Case has the advantage of being located in one of the largest cities with only one medical school. There are numerous affiliated hospitals, and almost all patients from every SES and with varied diseases are treated. The University Hospital has an academic atmosphere; many unusual cases and indigent patients are found there. The VA Hospital is short-staffed, so students learn the "nuts and bolts of medicine" here. Cleveland Metropolitan General Hospital serves an indigent population. There are various other hospitals, but those listed above are among the ones that students go to most often.

It is not difficult to locate housing in the area of the school, and much of it is within easy walking distance. Most students live in apartments, with the average cost of a one-bedroom apartment $275 per month.

ACADEMICS

Students do not recommend any particular science courses to premeds, with the possible exception of biochemistry or cell biology.

PHYSICAL ENVIRONMENT

Chicago Medical School moved into new buildings only a few years ago. The teaching facilities are brand new, and a teaching hospital is being built and will be completed in two years. There is a weight room in the school, but for other facilities, such as a gym and a pool, students go to the VA Hospital, which is only a mile away. Chicago Medical School is located in a suburban area near a golf course (which costs $5 per year to use). Students find that they are exposed to a very wide spectrum of both patients and cases through the school's affiliated hospitals.

Housing is easy to locate. The prices vary depending on where you wish to live. The school does not have its own student housing, but many students use a nearby college dormitory that is very inexpensive, costing about $160 per month. This living arrangement is preferred over living in apartments because of cost, but most students live off campus in apartments that generally range from $300 to $500 per month.

ACADEMICS

Volume, not content, is what makes the work load so much greater at this school. All exams are computer graded and are "board type." Students find that exams are graded fairly but not always made up fairly. Students are evaluated by a letter-grade system, and competition for A's (which in most classes less than 10 percent of students receive) is fierce. Several students here had to reevaluate what "good grades" means. However, a great number of students get B's, and the vast majority of students pass their courses. Students recommend taking "anything that will give you a jump on what's to come," including biochemistry, physiology, histology, and genetics.

As for study methods for succeeding at the Chicago Medical School, one student said the following: "I wouldn't [recommend any study methods]—if there is anything that I've learned, it's that everyone must discover what is the best method **for them**. I had the greatest difficulty when I tried to learn by someone else's **"foolproof method."** Consider the first year one big self-experiment and don't be afraid to try something else if you're not satisfied with the results from the method(s) that you've already tried." Another student did recommend studying material in detail early in the course because this way you will maintain a good "data base" for the later material, which is additive.

Students here are very complimentary of the faculty and administration, which, many say, "bend over backwards to do anything to help you." The student/faculty relationship is described as "intimate and personal" with many professors and deans willing to meet with students without appointments. There are excellent opportunities for student research, including a summer fellowship between first and second years in which several students participate. Chicago Medical School has worked towards increasing the number of electives that its students can choose from during their four years. Elective courses include medical jurisprudence, alcoholism, biostatistics, geriatrics, nutrition, and preventive medicine.

FINANCIAL

Loans (all types including HEAL) are considered a necessity for students who are not sponsored by either parents or spouses. The total cost for the first year will be about $27,000 primarily due to the cost of tuition. There are some work opportunities for students and their spouses offered by the school, but students advise against working while attending this medical school.

SOCIAL LIFE

Diverse. This is the first word that students here use to describe their class, which is one-third New York students, one-third West Coast students, and one-third Midwest students. Students describe themselves as "a normal group of people with not many gunners." There are many social gatherings, including barbecues, movies during the week, and parties on the weekend.

COMMENTS: A student here added the following observation about her medical school: "One very positive aspect of CMS is the strength, influence, and involvement of our student government. Our opinions are definitely listened to; we have fairly open access to our administrators, and direct lines of communication with all levels of our medical school."

COLUMBIA UNIVERSITY
College of Physicians and Surgeons
630 West 168th Street   /   New York, New York 10032

LOCATION: Urban/Big City

AGE OF SCHOOL: 221 Years

CONTROL: Private

AMCAS **MEMBER:** No

SIZE OF CLASS: 150

PERCENT WOMEN IN CLASS: 35

PERCENT MINORITIES IN CLASS: 15

AVERAGE STUDENT EXPENDITURE: $$$ (Both in-state and nonresident)

M.D.-Ph.D.: Yes—anatomy, biochemistry, chemistry, epidemiology, human genetics and development, mathematical statistics, microbiology, nutrition, pathology, pharmacology, physiology, and psychology; also available through Medical Scientists Training Program

NBME **Part I:** Passing score required for graduation

NBME **Part II:** Passing score required for graduation

Support services are available for disabled students through the Office of Disabled Student Services, the Office of Equal Opportunity and Affirmative Action, and the President's Advisory Committee on the Handicapped for the Health Sciences.

PHYSICAL ENVIRONMENT

Columbia University College of Physicians and Surgeons is housed in Columbia-Presbyterian Medical Center in the midst of a lower SES area of New York City. Columbia-Presbyterian is currently undergoing extensive renovations, and the school is planning the construction of "Audubon Park," which will house the first bio-industrial park in New York City. Columbia's basic sciences facilities are outstanding, and students have access to audiovisual playback equipment, preview rooms, and computerized bibliographies including MEDLARS. Columbia-Presbyterian and the Health Sciences Library will be part of a pilot project for the development of an Integrated Academic Information System.

Columbia has phenomenal clinical facilities that include affiliations with eight teaching sites. The major hospital site for medical students is Columbia-Presbyterian, which has an excellent nursing staff, advanced technology, and a wide range of patients with excellent opportunities for observation of complex medical cases. Others include the New York State Psychiatric Hospital, considered one of the best mental health facilities in New York; Mary Imogene Bassett Hospital, a well-run rural facility in Cooperstown, New York; Harlem Hospital Center, also well staffed and with good facilities; and Helen Hayes Hospital, a rehabilitation center known for its advances in the treatment of bone disease.

Students find the area around the medical school to be "a lot safer than it looks or is rumored to be." A sizable number of students, particularly first year, live in Bard Hall, which was recently renovated and costs students about $3100 for the year. There are numerous athletic facilities available in Bard Hall, including a basketball court, a swimming pool, a Universal Gym, a weight room, and two squash courts.

ACADEMICS

One student comments about the Columbia faculty, "They are the shining stars of both the basic and clinical sciences. Just look at the amount of research grants that the faculty at this school get. It's astounding!" Students agree that both the administration and the faculty make a concerted effort to help students, although at times some faculty have been known to be difficult to reach. Competition for grades (Honors/Pass/Fail) is felt by most students, but as one man says, "When push comes to shove, we all are willing to help each other out."

Students recommend having a sound foundation in biochemistry, histology, and genetics, as well as good communication and writing skills, before attending this school. There are excellent opportunities for student research, which is actively encouraged by the faculty.

The first two years at Columbia are primarily occupied with basic sciences and introduction to clinical skills beginning during the second semester of the second year and culminating in a four-week clerkship. The third year is mostly required clinical courses, and the fourth year offers numerous opportunities for individualized instruction and electives, including opportunities to study the delivery of health care in several foreign countries in conjunction with the School of Public Health.

FINANCIAL

Columbia will cost students approximately $23,000 for the first year. The financial aid office at this school is considered excellent and makes every attempt humanly possible to obtain aid for students. It is not recommended that students work during the school year because of the great demand of the course load.

SOCIAL LIFE

Columbia College of Physicians and Surgeons has one of the most organized and well-run student activities organizations in the country, which is known as P&S. P&S sponsors a diverse offering of clubs and activities, including parties, advocacy groups, film series, exercise groups, AMSA, American Medical Women's Association, the Bard Hall Players (theatrical group), and wine tasting. Besides the organized student activities, students have unlimited opportunities for social, cultural, and entertainment opportunities in New York City. Many students at this school tend to have gone to a relatively small number of the same schools (i.e., the Ivy League has a very high representation here), but students are also very diverse, talented, and caring.

COMMENTS: Columbia offers the best of everything to its students, with the possible exception of its location. The school has phenomenal clinical sites, an unbeatable faculty, and a lively and intensely self-motivated student body.

CORNELL UNIVERSITY
Medical School
1300 York Avenue / New York, New York 10021

LOCATION: Urban/Big City
AGE OF SCHOOL: 90 Years
CONTROL: Private
AMCAS **MEMBER:** Yes
CLASS SIZE: 101
PERCENT WOMEN IN CLASS: 38

PERCENT MINORITIES IN CLASS: 16

AVERAGE STUDENT EXPENDITURE: $$$ (Both in-state and nonresident)

M.D.-Ph.D.: Yes—with Cornell Graduate School of Medical Sciences and Sloan-Kettering Division of Graduate School of Medical Sciences— biochemistry, biophysics, cell and developmental biology, developmental therapy, genetics, immunology, microbiology, molecular biology, neurobiology and behavior, pathology, pharmacology, physiology, and virology; also, M.D.-Ph.D. available through Medical Scientist Training Program in conjunction with the Rockefeller Institute

NBME **Part I:** Optional

NBME **Part II:** Optional

PHYSICAL ENVIRONMENT

Going to medical school on the Upper East Side of Manhattan can offer students distinct advantages. Two major advantages Cornell Medical School affords its students are a relatively safe environment, particularly when compared to most New York schools, and reasonably priced and very livable housing across the street from the large stone complex where students take their basic sciences.

There are athletic facilities including a gym and a weight room in Olin Hall, and a swimming pool at the 54th Street Gym. The average cost for rooms is $210 per month in Olin Hall, an excellent housing facility for single first-year students. Upperclassmen and married students are able to live in two other nearby facilities: Livingston-Farrand Apartments and Lasdon House, in which students pay about $260 per month each for sharing their apartment.

Cornell medical students rotate out of some of the finest clinical sites in the country, including New York Hospital; Memorial Sloan-Kettering Cancer Center, one of the foremost centers for cancer research in the country; Rockefeller University; and the Hospital for Special Surgery. Students are exposed to a wide variety of SES patients and cases through this combination of clinical facilities.

ACADEMICS

The New Curriculum which Cornell began about three years ago enhanced students' opportunities for research, taking electives, and small-group learning, as well as improved the transition from basic sciences to clinical instruction. Through this program, classroom time was cut. This allows students to take between two and four half-days a week for electives, including research with the option of receiving the M.D. with Honors degree in Research. Introduction to Clinical Years is a new course that was designed to ease the transition from basic sciences to clinical exposure.

It is recommended that students take biochemistry, histology, and a computer course before attending this medical school. Studying with a partner, outlining lectures, and obtaining old tests is recommended for academic success. There is moderate competition for grades among students, although it is discouraged by the administration.

Students are able to use Macintosh computers in conjunction with Clinicopathological Conferences, which center on case histories of interest. The faculty here are highly accessible, very research oriented, and concerned with student needs.

FINANCIAL

The average first-year student will spend about $23,500 at this school. The financial aid office discourages the use of HEAL loans and attempts to get lower interest loans for students if at all possible. There are limited opportunities for work/study during the school year. There are many medically-related jobs available during the summer.

SOCIAL LIFE

Students at this school have numerous organizations and activities, including the Medical Student Excecutive Council which serves as a liason between students and the administration, the Student Research Society, AMSA, the American Medical Women's Association, Phi Delta Epsilon, and Students for Equal Opportunity in Medicine, an active minority organization.

COMMENTS: Cornell is a topnotch medical school with a flexible curriculum, a strong faculty, and a good location. Students at this school have the opportunity to see a wide variety of patients in outstanding clinical facilities. This is a particularly good medical school for those students interested in conducting research.

CREIGHTON UNIVERSITY
School of Medicine
2500 California Street / Omaha, Nebraska 68131

LOCATION: Urban/Medium-Sized City

AGE OF SCHOOL: 96 Years

CONTROL: Private

AMCAS **MEMBER:** Yes

CLASS SIZE: 110

PERCENT WOMEN IN CLASS: 25

PERCENT MINORITIES IN CLASS: 10

AVERAGE STUDENT EXPENDITURE: $$$ (Both in-state and nonresident)

M.D.-Ph.D.: Yes—anatomy, biochemistry, microbiology, and physiology

NBME **Part I:** Passing score required for promotion

NBME **Part II:** Optional

PHYSICAL ENVIRONMENT

Creighton University School of Medicine is a complex made up of three modern brick buildings. The school is located on the undergraduate campus, so there is easy access to athletic facilities. Creighton medical school is near downtown Omaha in an older part of town that is undergoing renovation. There are plenty of apartments close to the campus. A single apartment costs about $320 per month whereas a double runs about $350 per month. The area surrounding the school is relatively safe.

Students rotate through several hospitals, including Creighton Memorial St. Joseph Hospital, which is the main affiliated hospital and which is being renovated. This facility serves an indigent population as well as middle SES patients. Surgery and medicine often rotate out of the VA hospital, which has a lot of older veterans. An addition has recently been added to the clinics, and students do a lot of their own "scut work" while here. Children's Memorial Hospital is a very well-run facility, and many students do their pediatric rotations through this hospital, which treats upper to middle SES patients. Through the course of their rotations, students are exposed to patients from practically all backgrounds and to a wide variety of cases.

ACADEMICS

Students recommend taking as many nonscience courses as possible while still getting an adequate science background. English, literature, history, business management, and psychology, as well as physiology and microbiology, are recommended for prospective students. At present, competition among students is very intense, but steps are being taken to alleviate this competition. Pharmacology and microbiology are considered to be among the most difficult courses.

Students feel that to succeed you "must put your time in." They recommend purchasing review books with outlines of the subject and books with practice questions. There is a mix of professors here ranging from excellent to fair, with almost all having extensive knowledge of their course work. However, some professors need improvement in their presentation of the material. There are chances for student research, but the student must make the effort to get involved.

FINANCIAL

Creighton School of Medicine costs approximately $22,000 per year. A small number of students utilize a state sponsorship program to pay their tuition. Considering the amount of work and the emotional stress they are under, students do not feel that it is possible to work while attending Creighton medical school.

SOCIAL LIFE

Most social activities at this school are initated on an individual basis; there are not a lot of organized group activities. There are school parties and intramural sports for students. The class is made up of a well-rounded group of people with diverse backgrounds.

COMMENTS: Creighton's curriculum offers students some opportunities for independent study and numerous extramural electives. The faculty is considered good, and the affiliated hospitals will provide the students with a "nice mix of patients and cases."

DARTMOUTH MEDICAL SCHOOL
Hanover, New Hampshire 03755

LOCATION: Rural/Small City

AGE OF SCHOOL: 191 Years

CONTROL: Private

AMCAS **MEMBER:** No

CLASS SIZE: 100

PERCENT WOMEN IN CLASS: 50

PERCENT MINORITIES IN CLASS: 10

AVERAGE STUDENT EXPENDITURE: $$$$ (Both in-state and nonresident)

M.D.-Ph.D.: Yes—biochemistry, bioengineering, pharmacology, and physiology

NBME **Part I:** Optional

NBME **Part II:** Optional

PHYSICAL ENVIRONMENT

Students at Dartmouth Medical School have nothing but glowing comments about the area surrounding their school. Dartmouth is situated in a beautiful and quite scenic area of New Hampshire. The medical school is housed in relatively modern red-brick buildings that are attractive and easily accessible to the older, ivy-covered undergraduate campus. The basic sciences lecture facilities are in very good condition. The clinical facilities at Mary Hitchcock Memorial Hospital are adequate. However, a new medical complex is projected to be built by 1992. The plan is to move the medical school out of Hanover once the new complex is completed.

Most nonacademic facilities are within easy walking distance, so lunch time is often used to go to the gym to work out. The rural environment is conducive to a number of outdoor activities. Facilities include running trails, an outdoor ice rink, a ski slope, a golf course, and many outdoor tennis courts. The area surrounding the school is considered safe, and students feel that is not necessary to bring a car to school.

It is not difficult to find suitable housing. There are some dormitory rooms currently available, but these are slowly being phased out.

The average cost of a one-bedroom apartment ranges from $260 to $350 per month in Sachem Village, which is graduate student housing. A one-bedroom apartment off campus in the vicinity of the school ranges from $150 to $300 per month. Apartments and shared houses are the most common form of housing. Students strongly recommend these living options over staying in an on-campus dorm room.

ACADEMICS

One student compares the first year of Dartmouth Medical School to a very rigorous premedical training program in which one completes all the science prerequisites in one year. It is recommended that students take humanities as undergraduates as well as cell biology and biochemistry, which some students are able to place out of, making their course load lighter. Economics was suggested because it teaches the allocation of scarce resources, including the delivery of health care.

Competition for good grades (grading system: Honors/Pass/Fail) has increased in recent years, although it is not what one might call intense. Anatomy is considered among the hardest courses due to the volume of material covered. Students stress preparing before classes. Listening to the lecture will be then an active process of thinking with the professor as material is covered rather than a passive process of simply taking notes. In the words of one first-year student, "Reviewing and repetition are also key. Study groups help tremendously—verbalizing forces you to realize what you do or do not know."

Students feel that the school could use more faculty. They find the faculty for the most part to be very caring about students. There are several famous professors among the faculty and they are accessible to students. The deans are very understanding about student needs and truly care about student issues and individual problems. There are some opportunities for student research, but these are not highly publicized. This school is more clinical than research oriented.

One program of considerable interest is the "offspring" of a course called Clinical Symposium. It is Family Medicine Longitudinal Elective, which provides students with firsthand exposure to the doctor-patient relationship as well as the chance to work with a doctor in family medicine. Clinical Symposium teaches interviewing skills in the biopsychosocial medicine model together with issues concerning the economics of medicine, social issues in medicine, and preventive medicine. Dartmouth students also have early patient exposure in psychiatry; they are allowed to interview a patient in a small group under the supervision of a psychologist or psychiatric resident.

There is a special Dartmouth-Brown Program under which 20 students study for their first two years at Dartmouth and finish their medical education at Brown, picking up a Brown medical degree. This program is excellent for those interested in gaining their basic sciences instruction in a more laid-back rural setting and their clinical training in an urban environment.

FINANCIAL

The cost of attending Dartmouth ranges from $25,000 to $28,000 for the first year. Many students have chosen to take military scholarships in order to pay for their medical education at Dartmouth. The financial aid office is highly regarded, and the school provides loans for students at lower rates than HEALs. There are some work/study jobs provided by the school, and students feel that working is possible.

SOCIAL LIFE

There are several social events scheduled for students at this school. "Liver Rounds" are monthly parties held at the school. Many students are active in intramural sports, and the second-year students do skits in February. A sizable number of medical students attended Dartmouth as undergraduates, and as one student says, "There's always someone who knows of a fraternity party over at the main campus."

COMMENTS: A major myth surrounding Dartmouth is that because it is a rural school, its students do not see enough patients. This is for the most part unfounded, and students feel they have ample exposure to patients. The construction of the new medical complex will make clinical training here even better. Dartmouth medical school attracts a varied group of students dedicated to excellence in medicine. This is an especially good program for students interested in family medicine.

DUKE UNIVERSITY
School of Medicine
Box 3710 / Durham, North Carolina 27710

LOCATION: Suburban/Small City

AGE OF SCHOOL: 58 Years

CONTROL: Private

AMCAS **MEMBER:** No

CLASS SIZE: 120

PERCENT WOMEN IN CLASS: 35

PERCENT MINORITIES IN CLASS: 2

AVERAGE STUDENT EXPENDITURE: $$$ (Both in-state and nonresident)

M.D.-Ph.D.: Yes—anatomy, biochemistry, biomedical engineering, computer science, genetics, microbiology, pathology, pharmacology, and physiology; also, combined M.D.-J.D. program with Duke Law School.

NBME **Part I:** Optional

NBME **Part II:** Optional

PHYSICAL ENVIRONMENT

Duke has beautiful gothic buildings situated in a seemingly suburban environment, although some students feel that Durham is a little too small to have suburbs. The medical school itself is located in the "old part" of the hospital known as Duke South. It is a relatively modern building with very modern lab facilities and a comfortable amphitheater for basic sciences classes. Most of the clinical year is spent in Duke North, which was opened in 1980 and is very modern. New construction is currently underway at the VA hospital and at Duke North, where wings for OB/GYN are being built.

Duke is affiliated with several outstanding hospitals. Duke Medical Center is well-staffed with IV teams. The facilities are modern (built in 1980) and up to date. The Durham VA Hospital is understaffed. Cape Fear Valley Hospital is a private hospital located in Fayetteville, N.C. Patients from this facility are generally of middle SES.

The medical school is in a safe area and is within walking distance of several facilities, ranging from a gym (five-minute walk), pools, and tennis courts to libraries. It is very easy to locate housing near the school and some housing, which is near the hospital, is provided for graduate students. Apartments are the most plentiful form of housing used by medical students, with housing costing $170 to $250 per month per person for a double room and $300 to $460 per month per person for a single room in an apartment.

ACADEMICS

Duke medical school has an interesting curriculum in which students finish their basic sciences during the first year. This gives students an opportunity to reflect on what they have learned during the second year, spent with patients. The third year is used by most students to conduct independent research, and many students choose basic sciences as topics for their research. Like most medical schools, Duke offers its students electives in the fourth year.

Several students compare the first year to drinking water from a fire hose, but practically all are ecstatic about having the opportunity for earlier entry into the clinic and the chance to conduct independent research.

Students recommend that premeds take biochemistry ("very important"), English composition and literature, art, history, and nonscience courses that you may not have a chance to take again. Exams are graded fairly. Competition is not intense because "everyone's pretty good about studying together and sharing any resources such as old exams." Duke grades are on a Pass/Fail/Honors system.

Gross anatomy and pharmacology are considered among the most challenging courses. One student recommends getting The Anatomy Coloring Book for anatomy. "Keep up!!" advises one woman who says that paying attention in class can help you save hours of studying time later. Professors care a great deal about students and help them learn the material in and out of the classroom. However, the Faculty Advising System is somewhat weak and is being improved at this time. Students spend between 4 and 6 hours a night studying.

FINANCIAL

Although Duke medical school provides more jobs for students than are taken, it is cautioned that even though working may be possible, it also could be psychologically difficult since it would leave no free time to relax. Loans are a must for most at Duke, with the first year averaging about $22,000 total. There is a high ratio (12 percent) of students on HPSP (Health Professsions Scholarship Program) scholarships.

SOCIAL LIFE

Duke medical students are bright, interesting, and diversified. There are many social events scheduled, including parties, dances, "Renewal of Systems" with faculty members, and a student-faculty show. Asked why he chose Duke, one student responded, "its reputation, the second year clinical rotations, and the location."

COMMENTS: There is no question that this school is an excellent place to spend your four years (or six for those interested in M.D.-Ph.D. programs) of medical school. The curriculum is innovative, and both students and faculty here are very enthusiastic and have a strong interest in both research and clinical medicine. Duke is actively recruiting qualified minority applicants, although there are currently very few minority students at this school.

EMORY UNIVERSITY
School of Medicine
1440 Clifton Road, N.E.   /   Atlanta, Georgia 30322

LOCATION: Suburban/Big City

AGE OF SCHOOL: 134 Years

CONTROL: Private

AMCAS **MEMBER:**   Yes

SIZE OF CLASS: 110

PERCENT WOMEN IN CLASS: 35

PERCENT MINORITIES IN CLASS: 5

AVERAGE STUDENT EXPENDITURE: $$$ (Both in-state and nonresident)

M.D.-Ph.D.:   Yes—biophysical chemistry, immunology, membrane biophysics, genetics, and neuroscience; also, M.D.-Master's of Public Health (M.P.H.) available

NBME **Part I:**   Passing score required for promotion

NBME **Part II:**   Student must record a score.

PHYSICAL ENVIRONMENT

Emory University School of Medicine consists of moderately aged buildings situated on a beautiful campus. There are a new gym, health sciences library, and student union. There is adequate lab space, and the laboratories are in good condition. The addition of the new library provides students with plenty of study space. There are extensive computer facilities and on-line services, including MEDLINE.

Emory has extensive hospital affiliations, including the University Hospital which houses both a psychiatric unit and an NIH-supported clinical research facilty. Grady Memorial Hospital is in fair condition, and most students rotate out of this facility, which treats a great deal of lower SES patients. The VA hospital is in very good condition; Crawford Long Memorial Hospital has "very advanced technology and a good nursing staff"; the Emory Clinic is a private partnership between the Emory medical faculty and "houses numerous specialists and treats many complex cases"; the Rehabilitation Center is a very good facility with much research currently underway; Yerkes Primate Research Center is an NIH-sponsored facility (one of seven in the country), and a new Ophthalmic Research Facility has recently been added to the center.

The school itself is located in a clean and relatively safe suburban part of Atlanta. Students recommend bringing a car if possible. Most students choose to live in moderately priced apartments costing from $250 to $350 per month. On-campus housing is also in the form of apartments, ranging from $242 to $292 per month. Athletic facilities are housed in the George Woodruff Physical Education Center and are accessible for medical students.

ACADEMICS

The courses are more demanding than undergraduate work due to the heavier volume of material covered. However, students find that the work is manageable. It is recommended that students take embryology, biochemistry, and histology before entering this school. Competition for good grades (grading system: A/B/C/D/E/F; S/U for electives) is present but not intense. As one student says, "People are conscious of the grades they are making."

Students recommend keeping up daily with class notes in order to succeed on exams. The faculty are interested in helping students and rarely require appointments to meet with them. Several opportunities for student research are provided by the school, with stipends for summer projects. Students selected this school for its reputation, faculty, and excellent clinical experience.

FINANCIAL

The total cost of attending Emory will be about $23,000 for the first year. Most students take out GSLs. Although working is not recommended during the second year, there are lab jobs available in the hospital.

SOCIAL LIFE

Emory is not only a "warm school in a warm setting," but it also gives its students plenty of chances to socialize outside the classroom. There are movies, concerts, plays, and intramural sports for students. Numerous student organizations, including Ad Hoc Productions, a student-organized group that puts on one major production per year; the Student National Medical Association for black medical students; and several honorary societies provide students with nonacademic outlets. About half of the students at Emory School of Medicine are from Georgia. Nonresidents must provide somewhat better academic records to be competitive with Georgia residents.

COMMENTS: Emory's strongest features are its location, clinical affiliations, and faculty. There are good opportunities for research, and several scholarships are awarded each year by the school, ranging from $500 to $5750. Emory is making a good effort to attract more minority applicants.

GEORGETOWN UNIVERSITY
School of Medicine
3900 Reservoir Road, N.W. / Washington, D.C. 20007

LOCATION: Suburban/Big City
AGE OF SCHOOL: 137 Years
CONTROL: Private (Religious affiliation: Catholic)
AMCAS **MEMBER:** Yes

SIZE OF CLASS: 200

PERCENT WOMEN IN CLASS: 30

PERCENT MINORITIES IN CLASS: 10

AVERAGE STUDENT EXPENDITURE: $$$$ (Both in-state and nonresident)

M.D.-Ph.D.:   Yes—anatomy, biochemistry, pathology, pharmacology, physiology, and biophysics

NBME **Part I:**   Optional

NBME **Part II:**   Optional

PHYSICAL ENVIRONMENT

Georgetown School of Medicine is housed in a very attractive facility that "has elements of both modern and classical architecture." One student describes the area surrounding Georgetown School of Medicine and the school itself: "These are the things you will NOT have to worry about: safety (it's in a wealthy, suburban neighborhood and there haven't been many incidents of people being bothered around the school at night), facilities (the library is excellent with great study aids, and there's plenty of space in the labs and the lecture halls), and finding reasonably priced housing near the school (there isn't any to speak of!)." Georgetown is located in a very affluent Washington suburb. It is easy to get to the undergraduate campus's athletic facilities, including a swimming pool, weight room, and gymnasium.

There is certainly no question that Georgetown's clinical facilities are among its biggest assets. Georgetown University Hospital, the major teaching facility, is made up of four components, including The Concentrated Care Center, an excellent facility for the acutely ill ("You have to see this place to believe it. The equipment is so modern."); The Lombardi Cancer Center, a newer building with extensive cancer research and treatment facilities; and The Gorman Building, with outstanding technological advances such as Gorman Auditorium in which each seat is equipped with a jack and stethophone for examination of the patient during clinical conferences. The school is affiliated with numerous health care facilities, including D.C. General, Fairfax Hospital, the National Naval Medical Center, and Walter Reed Army Hospital. Students are exposed to a great variety of both cases and patients through the combination of the school's clinical sites.

Finding suitable housing does pose something of a problem to students, particularly because the Georgetown area is a seller's market. A single room in a house costs between $300 and $500 per month, one-bedroom apartments average between $500 to $800 per month, and a two-bedroom apartment runs between $900 to $1500 per month. *Important Tip:* Students recommend obtaining housing in Arlington, Virginia, which is not far from Georgetown and is much less expensive (although still not cheap), with one-bedroom apartments costing between $250 and $400 per month. Students should begin looking for housing as soon as possible ("at least a month and a half before the start of school").

The Georgetown University Transportation Society (GUTS) is a bus that takes students to parts of Washington and Virginia. Students can opt for a meal plan through the Darnall and New South cafeterias or through the highly recommended Caduceus cafeteria, which is housed in the Medical/Dental Building.

ACADEMICS

Georgetown students recommend taking courses in biochemistry, histology, and computers before attending their medical school. The majority of the basic sciences exams are multiple-choice. Competition among students is "present, but it serves as a healthy stimulus rather than creating an overwhelming feeling of pressure." Georgetown has an innovative and somewhat flexible curriculum that introduces students to clinical medicine (Introduction to Clinical Medicine is a four-semester course) early in their education, allows for electives throughout all four years, and provides opportunities for research and independent study.

Students comment that some of the faculty members could be "a little more approachable." But, overall the faculty is considered to be "interesting, good teachers who are interested in more than our [the students'] committing Kreb's Cycle to memory. They want us to know how to apply what we learn to medicine and everyday life (if possible)."

FINANCIAL

Georgetown will cost students a total of approximately $26,000 for the first year. The financial aid office is adequate at this school, and most students take out numerous loans, including GSL, NDSL, and

HEAL. There are some work opportunities offered by the school during the year, but students advise against working, particularly during the first year, because of the work load and the time necessary to get adjusted.

SOCIAL LIFE

Students here believe having an active social life is an important component of medical education. The school is close to the White House, the Air and Space Museum, the Library of Congress, and the National Gallery of Art. Georgetown medical students have an active voice in what goes on in their school and meet with the faculty and administration on a regular basis to dicuss student issues. The class tends to be made up of upper to middle SES students with a few older students.

COMMENTS: Georgetown is a mecca for medical students. The only drawbacks are the high cost of living near the school and the high cost of attending this outstanding medical school. The curriculum allows students a certain degree of freedom, the faculty are very good, the clinical sites are not only numerous but also exemplary, and there are abundant opportunities for research.

HAHNEMANN UNIVERSITY
School of Medicine
Broad and Vine Streets / Philadelphia, Pennsylvania 19102

LOCATION: Urban/Big City

AGE OF SCHOOL: 140 Years

CONTROL: Private

AMCAS MEMBER: Yes

CLASS SIZE: 170

PERCENT WOMEN IN CLASS: 33

PERCENT MINORITIES IN CLASS: 16

AVERAGE STUDENT EXPENDITURE: $$$ (Both in-state and nonresident)

M.D.-Ph.D.: Yes—offered in numerous academic areas including most basic sciences; also, combined program with undergraduate and combined D.D.S.-M.D. program available

NBME **Part I:** Students must pass for promotion to third year.

NBME **Part II:** Students must pass for graduation.

PHYSICAL ENVIRONMENT

Hahnemann University School of Medicine is located in a modern 19-story building. The main lecture halls and classrooms are located on the first four floors. The Allied Health Building, which is next to the medical school, has a fully equipped Nautilus room, and there is a YMCA five blocks away. The campus bookstore, game rooms, library, and financial aid offices are all located within the medical school building.

The laboratory and classroom facilities at Hahnemann are in good condition. The school has a variety of very adequate clinical sites including the Hahnemann Ambulatory Health Services Center; the University Hospital, which has an excellent nursing staff and up-to-date equipment; the Cardiovascular Research Institute; and several other affiliated hospitals. The school is located in Center City in Philadelphia in what students considered a "semi-safe area." Most students live in dormitories, but off-campus housing is also available. Dorm suites and one-bedroom apartments in the area of the school go for between $350 and $400 per month.

ACADEMICS

Students recommend taking biochemistry ("It is important to have a basic foundation"), histology, psychology, and human developmental biology ("not frogs and chickens"). Competition for grades is "all but nonexistent" with Hahnemann's Pass/Fail grading system. Study methodologies for success at this school include using study groups to pick up information that your classmates might have learned that passed you by during the lecture, very strong organizational skills, and breaks between studying because the normal attention span prohibits learning information in large "blocks of time."

Students find that the faculty here are excellent, but one woman comments that there are not enough of them. Most students agree that tutoring and counseling are available for students when the need arises. Hahnemann is a research-oriented medical school, and there are numerous opportunities for student involvement in faculty research.

FINANCIAL

Hahnemann will cost first-year students a total of approximately $23,000. The school offers some low-interest loans and a limited number of scholarships. Most students take out GSLs and many use HEAL loans as well as support from parents and spouses. After the first year students find that it is possible to work part-time, and there are jobs in the library, hospital, and doing research.

SOCIAL LIFE

There are some social events at this school, including parties and organized trips. The class is diverse and there is a very good support system for minority students. Hahnemann medical students are generally "laid-back" and do not overreact to the pressures of medical school as much as do other medical students.

COMMENTS: Hahnemann is a research-oriented school, but students here find the clinical faculty to be somewhat better communicators of information. The school has adequate clinical affiliations and a passable location that is near very good cultural and entertainment areas.

HARVARD MEDICAL SCHOOL
25 Shattuck Street / Boston, Massachusetts 02115

LOCATION: Urban/Big City

AGE OF SCHOOL: 206 Years

CONTROL: Private

AMCAS **MEMBER:** No

CLASS SIZE: 165

PERCENT WOMEN IN CLASS: 37

PERCENT MINORITIES IN CLASS: 15

AVERAGE STUDENT EXPENDITURE: $$$ (Both in-state and nonresident)

M.D.-Ph.D.: Yes—available in conjunction with a full complement of academic areas, including basic sciences, engineering, and social sciences; also available through Medical Scientist Training Program in conjunction with Massachusetts Institute of Technology

NBME **Part I:** Passing score required for promotion

NBME **Part II:** Passing score required for graduation

PHYSICAL ENVIRONMENT

Premedical students with the preconceived notion that Harvard Medical School looks like a castle or some other romantic ideal may be disillusioned after setting eyes on the large and somewhat imposing stone quadrangle of buildings which makes up this highly respected institution of medical learning. These same students will be relieved to know that inside these buildings, amidst the heavy construction, both the romantic and practical ideals of medicine are very much alive. Each room in the older part of the school, from the "old amphitheater" to the tiny elevator that transports students to a fascinating museum showcasing advances in medicine, exudes history.

But, students here are equally proud of the newly constructed laboratories and classrooms that are equipped with the latest technological equipment. The Countway Library of Medicine, one of the largest such libraries in the country, is also the home of the prestigious *New England Journal of Medicine*. Students have the use of state-of-the-art computers to stimulate various medical conditions. One of the many benefits of attending Harvard is the proximity of the school to its affiliated hospitals.

Virtually all of Harvard's clinical sites are considered to be among the best hospitals in the United States. Students are exposed to an enormous variety of patients and complex cases through rotations at Beth Israel Hospital, Brigham and Womens Hospital, and Massachusetts General Hospital, which has the latest medical technology available.

The area around the school is considered relatively safe, and there are security guards in most of the buildings. Most first-year students choose to live in Vanderbilt Hall, which is right across the street from the medical school. The cost for this accomodation is between $280 and $360 per month. After the first year, many students move out into and share apartments costing between $275 and $350 per month. Students have easy access to athletic facilities, including a gymnasium.

ACADEMICS

Harvard's curriculum is both traditional and innovative, consisting of three main programs. The Health Science and Technology Program is sponsored in conjunction with the Massachusetts Institute of Technology (reached by shuttle bus). Students in this program pay close attention to quantitative sciences, including bioengineering, biophysics, and chemical sciences. The students also have ample interaction with patients during the third and fourth years, at which time they are involved in clinical clerkships. These students are also responsible for the presentation of a thesis.

The Oliver Wendell Holmes Society is the newest program at Harvard and is based largely on small-group learning through application of scientific information to individual case histories and independent research. The strengths of this program are its facilitating research methodology and integration of clinical, basic, and social sciences. Students taught using the traditional method of medical instruction, in which students take notes and listen to and read about information and research findings highlighted for them by a professor, may have the initial advantage of retaining more information in the short term. But, it is hoped that students taught using this innovative approach will be better off in the long term, with a more thorough understanding of the information they themselves have found, and have a better ability to integrate and apply their knowledge. This program offers students greater freedom to choose from areas of personal interest relevant to medicine.

The Classic Curriculum, which encompases most of the class, also allows for a good deal of freedom beginning in the first year. This approach relies far more heavily on the "traditional" methodology of medical instruction, whereby students learn through the research findings of faculty members and study from the class syllabus. Beginning during the 1987–88 session students in the Classic Curriculum will have part of their course work (the unit entitled The Body) taught in the same manner as the Oliver Wendell Holmes Society. Students in the Classic Curriculum find that there is minimal competition for grades (Excellent/Pass/Fail).

The faculty is praised by all students, as summed up by one man: "They really go out of their way to find interesting lecturers, present the most current research, and entertain students' suggestions and ideas. They make it [medical school] a dynamic learning experience." It is recommended that students have a solid foundation in the basic sciences before attending this school. Courses recommended include biochemistry, histology, writing, and communications.

FINANCIAL

The first year of Harvard Medical School will cost a total of about $25,000. The school's financial aid office is considered outstanding, and there are numerous scholarships and loans administered by Harvard. Some students work in laboratory and hospital jobs, although it is recommended that students refrain from working during the first year.

SOCIAL LIFE

Harvard Medical School is a bus ride away from the heart of Boston, which has limitless cultural, entertainment, and shopping areas. There are student organizations, intramural sports, and parties. What is most impressive about the medical students is not their extreme academic prowess (which is self-evident upon talking with them) but rather their openness to new ideas and their candor.

COMMENTS: If you noticed an excessive use of superlatives in the description of this medical school, you have begun to understand just some of the reasons why this is one of the top medical schools in the nation, if not the world. Harvard is a "name school" that did not sit on its laurels but instead used its outstanding reputation to build an even better school with a new and innovative curriculum that is leading the way in medical education, outstanding clinical and basic sciences facilities, faculty who are virtually unparalleled, and a dynamic, highly intelligent, self-motivated, and research-oriented student body.

JEFFERSON MEDICAL COLLEGE
1025 Walnut Street / Philadelphia, Pennsylvania 19107

LOCATION: Urban/Big City

AGE OF SCHOOL: 164 Years

CONTROL: Private (With state subsidy)

AMCAS **MEMBER:** Yes

CLASS SIZE: 223

PERCENT WOMEN IN CLASS: 40

PERCENT MINORITIES IN CLASS: 5

AVERAGE STUDENT EXPENDITURE: $$$ (Both in-state and nonresident)

M.D.-Ph.D.: Yes—anatomy, biochemistry, microbiology, pathology, pharmacology, and physiology

NBME **Part I:** Passing grade required for promotion

NBME **Part II:** Passing grade required for graduation

PHYSICAL ENVIRONMENT

Jefferson Medical College is made up of both old and new buildings situated in a very clean and well-guarded campus. The school is ". . . large enough, yet still contained." The gym is downstairs from the medical school classrooms. Jefferson medical school is located in the heart of Philadelphia, which offers students an endless variety of cultural and social activities. A major issue about this school is the safety. Although the area surrounding Jefferson is not particularly safe, there is a new "beefed-up" security system being introduced. Students believe that precautions must be taken for safety, such as walking in groups or using the escort service, but the problem is not as bad as it has been made out to be.

One of the major drawing points of Jefferson is its numerous hospital sites. The school is affiliated with hospitals in Pennsylvania, New Jersey, and Delaware. The library has a floor that is open 24 hours a day for late-night studiers. The basic sciences labs are both convenient and clean.

Finding housing is easy because the school provides three on-campus housing facilities. Two of the on-campus residences are apartment complexes, and one is a dormitory, all of which are considered to be expensive but competitive with Philadelphia housing costs. Apartments in the area of the school range from $150 to $500 per month. Many students elect to live in one of the five fraternity houses near the school.

ACADEMICS

The first thing a medical student will mention about Jefferson is its numerical grading system. "It's really not that bad," says one man. Students here are quick to point out that "gunners" are present at most medical schools and that grades are a measure of self-achievement. Interestingly, students find that those students groveling for grades are usually at the upper end of the curve. Competition for grades is present but is not as intense as might be expected.

It is recommended that students take ethics and basic statistics (to understand scientific papers) before entering. Physiology and pharmacology are difficult courses. For physiology, students stress studying the "overall picture" before concentrating on details, so there will be something to relate the facts to. For pharmacology, it is best to memorize the drugs, indications, effects, and side effects. Group studying is vital for success in gross anatomy. In general, it is helpful to take advantage of the student note service, attend as many lectures as possible, and read all recommended texts. Tests are primarily multiple-choice.

The school is not overly concerned with research, although there are opportunities for student research. Jefferson's emphasis is primarily on clinical instruction, and this is evidenced by the number of positive remarks students have about their clinical instruction.

FINANCIAL

The cost for attending Jefferson Medical College is about $24,000. Loans are considered a "must" for most students. Jefferson does award both scholarships and low-interest loans. There is also a work/study program for those who are eligible. It is difficult to work while attending with the exception of working as a phlebotomist on weekends at area hospitals.

SOCIAL LIFE

Students at Jefferson have a myriad of social possibilities because of the several active fraternities at the school. There are intramural sports, TGIF dances, lectures, banquets, and fund-raisers.

COMMENTS: The hospital facilities and clinical instruction at Jefferson are very good. Students at this school are very hardworking; many have taken time off prior to entering medical school. The school is working very hard to attract more minority students.

JOHNS HOPKINS UNIVERSITY
School of Medicine

720 Rutland Avenue / Baltimore, Maryland 21205

LOCATION: Urban/Big City

AGE OF SCHOOL: 95 Years

CONTROL: Private

AMCAS **MEMBER:** No

CLASS SIZE: 80

PERCENT WOMEN IN CLASS: 33

PERCENT MINORITIES IN CLASS: 10

AVERAGE STUDENT EXPENDITURE: $$$ (Both in-state and nonresident)

M.D.-Ph.D.: Yes—available in conjunction with numerous basic sciences as well as biomedical engineering; also available through Medical Scientist Training Program. A combined 5-year program B.A.-M.D. is possible for students who have completed two years of college work.

NBME **Part I:** Optional

NBME **Part II:** Optional

PHYSICAL ENVIRONMENT

Johns Hopkins University School of Medicine is housed in a modern and recently renovated preclinical building and hospital. The school is located in what students refer to as a "semi-safe area." Perhaps *ghetto* is too strong a word, but the area is not particularly safe. However, there is a security van that picks up students, and the area is heavily patrolled and guarded.

Johns Hopkins students rotate out of some of the finest hospitals in the nation. Johns Hopkins Hospital is recently renovated and is in excellent condition. The students treat both indigent patients, primarily in the emergency room, and middle to upper SES patients who are referred in from out of town. Many alcoholism and AIDS cases are treated in this hospital. Francis Scott Key Hospital two miles away, is not a modern facility, but it will be torn down in 1989 and replaced by a $500-million research and development facility. Wyman Park Hospital, North Charles Hospital, and Good Samaritan Hospital are private community hospitals and are also excellent clinical facilities.

Housing is not difficult to locate in the area of the school, and for the most part, it is inexpensive. Row houses, cheap and spacious, cost students $210 per month for their share of the rent. A one-bedroom apartment runs about $250 per month. Reed Hall is the student dormitory, and it is not in the safest neighborhood. There are suites and single rooms in this facility. Johns Hopkins also has promoted the development of condos in the vicinity of the medical school, and several students take advantage of these inexpensive housing opportunities. It is a very good idea to have a car at Johns Hopkins.

ACADEMICS

The "Hopkins tradition" is very strong at this school. The school thinks of itself as a family, especially within individual departments. Prospective students should expect an intense environment, the result of having many strong-willed (not to mention brilliant) minds assembled in one place. Biochemistry is recommended for prospective students as well as English and philosophy. Competition for good grades (grading system: A/B/C/D/F) is definitely present. The hardest courses encountered by students are microbiology and immunology. Students here are encouraged to "think" rather than to simply memorize material. As a result, most exams are comprised largely of essays.

The faculty are superb and are willing to teach, although some students complain that they are a bit too research oriented. As you might guess, there are ample opportunities for research at this school. Most faculty attempt to teach material relevant to medical students and not just trivia. Says one student, "There is an expert here on just about everything." Study methods that work for students include studying with groups of students. One man states, "Fellow students are a great source of knowledge. I am always amazed at how much I can learn by trying to answer questions fellow students have raised. Having so many stimulating minds in one place is good for all of us."

FINANCIAL

A year at Johns Hopkins medical school will cost a single student about $25,000. Students take advantage of all loans possible and feel it is possible to work, but not many hours. There are lab jobs at Johns Hopkins in the summer (three months for $1250). Some students also work at the blood bank, and there is work/study provided by the school. Some subinternships offer payment to students. One student recommended living at home to save money if at all possible.

SOCIAL LIFE

There are several social events scheduled for students including the Dean's Fund Party, Christmas parties, and end-of-the-year parties. It is easy to find a few good friends at this school. The class is diverse and from many geographic areas and colleges.

COMMENT: This is certainly one of the top medical schools in the nation for more reasons than the large amount of money being allocated for faculty research. The student body is bright and articulate, and students are encouraged to look beyond rote answers to complex medical problems. The hospital sites are excellent and provide a diverse patient population with a variety of cases. Much like the school's philosophy, the students here think of themselves as a family, a rather intense and highly motivated family of future physicians.

LOMA LINDA UNIVERSITY
School of Medicine
Loma Linda, California 92350

LOCATION: Small Town
AGE OF SCHOOL: 78 Years

CONTROL: Private (Religious affiliation: Seventh-Day Adventist)

AMCAS **MEMBER:** Yes

CLASS SIZE: 150

PERCENT WOMEN IN CLASS: 30

PERCENT MINORITIES IN CLASS: 5

AVERAGE STUDENT EXPENDITURE: $$$ (Both in-state and nonresident)

M.D.-Ph.D.: Yes; Available in conjunction with several basic sciences

NBME **Part I:** Passing grade required for promotion.

NBME **Part II:** Passing grade required for graduation.

PHYSICAL ENVIRONMENT

Loma Linda's medical center is very impressive. The school is made up of several predominantly modern-style buildings. Athletic and campus facilities are a five-minute walk away. There is planned renovation and there may be a consolidation of La Sierra campus with Loma Linda. This consolidation includes plans for many new buildings and replacement of an existing gymnasium.

Both clinical and basic sciences facilities are very adequate. For students who wish to have part of their instruction in Los Angeles, 12 students per year can elect to spend their clinical years at White Memorial Hospital in East Los Angeles. Students complain that the school is culturally isolated and in a heavy smog area.

Finding housing does not seem to be a problem for most. Inexpensive housing is provided by the university, and the payment plan can be billed through the accounts office. An average one-bedroom apartment costs about $250 per month plus utilities. Students prefer to live in apartments and shared houses.

ACADEMICS

Loma Linda recently acquired a new female dean. There is talk of Loma Linda breaking up the traditional basic sciences instruction into small-group discussions that are problem-oriented. However, this change is coming about slowly, and students find that there is still what feels like a never-ending lecture. Students recommend taking Spanish, religion, ethics, sociology, psychology, microbiology, and computer and business courses. There does not appear to be intense competition for grades, which are Pass/Fail (students are ranked), although competition is far greater the first two years than the last two.

Loma Linda has a freshman study building, which students find helpful for group studying. It is also advised that students go over old tests and review the day's notes the same evening if possible. Anatomy, pharmacology, and microbiology are considered to be among the hardest preclinical courses here. Faculty are considered supportive and helpful, but some students find them too "cosmologically" concerned. "The reference to philosophy is always stated. However, it should be noted that is a stated goal for the faculty."

There are research opportunities that are in the developmental stages. Many students do summer and elective research projects, and stipends are available for summer research. The school is known for its work in international health and emphasis on spirituality and preventive medicine. However, the training is not much different from other medical schools, with the exception of some required religion courses.

FINANCIAL

The average student spends about $23,000 for the first year at Loma Linda medical school. Both scholarships and are loans are available to students. It is not advised to work while attending, but the school does provide phlebotomy jobs for students in the medical center.

SOCIAL LIFE

Official functions at Loma Linda medical school are "very conservative." The social structure of Adventism precludes a "party" atmosphere. However, there are Halloween parties, banquets, and Christmas concerts. There are also weekend retreats to the mountains. The social events are often religious, as might be expected from a school that is religiously affiliated and oriented.

COMMENTS: In general, students at this school are mostly Seventh-Day Adventists. The majority of students are conservative. However, one student believes there are many "clandestine progessives" in the midst of the conservative student body. Overall, the students are both compassionate and intelligent, with a keen interest in medicine.

MARSHALL UNIVERSITY
School of Medicine
Huntington, West Virginia 25701

LOCATION: Medium-Sized City

AGE OF SCHOOL: 16 Years

CONTROL: Public/State

AMCAS MEMBER: Yes

CLASS SIZE: 50

PERCENT WOMEN IN CLASS: 33

PERCENT MINORITIES IN CLASS: N/A

AVERAGE STUDENT EXPENDITURE: $ (Both in-state and nonresident)

M.D.-Ph.D.: No

NBME Part I: Passing score required for promotion

NBME Part II: Passing score required for graduation

PHYSICAL ENVIRONMENT

Marshall University School of Medicine is a new facility, less than seven years old, with a modern basic sciences building. The school is located on the grounds of the VA hospital. The VA is old, but it is slated for expansion and renovation in 1989. There are two modern community hospitals, as well as an older mental hospital that is being renovated.

The Medical Education Building is about a 15-minute drive from the downtown campus. The clinics are on the main campus during the last two years of instruction, so the gym, the pool, and the racquetball courts are especially accessible during these years. The school is currently building an MRI (Magnetic Resonance Imaging) facility, and a new clinic for all services should be built in the next three years.

The medical school is out of town, with a nearby golf course, houses, and apartments, and is relatively safe. Although there is no dorm living, finding suitable housing does not seem to be a problem. A three-bedroom house costs between $275 and $400 per month. An average two-bedroom apartment ranges from $180 to $200 per month.

ACADEMICS

Students feel that the course load is far more demanding, with a heavier volume, than their undergraduate schedules. Students recommend taking biochemistry, histology, genetics, and statistics before attending this medical school. There is not much competition for grades "unless you want to be #1 in your class." Histology, biochemistry, and neuroanatomy are considered to be among the hardest basic sciences courses.

Students believe that "studying at a steady rate" is an effective method for succeeding when coupled with taking time off as needed to refresh your attitude. One man recommends studying class notes and using texts only for reference. There is an excellent student-faculty relationship at this school, due in part to the fact that it is a small school with only 50 students per class. All faculty are accessible for questions and extra help.

There are many opportunities in most departments for research, along with several stipends. Students selected this school based on the faculty, friendly atmosphere, small class size, and new facilities.

FINANCIAL

Marshall medical school costs the average single first-year student about $10,000; for nonresidents, $13,000. Loans are available and many students take advantage of them, but the tuition for the school is relatively low when compared to other medical schools. It is possible to work while attending Marshall, and first- and second-year students are offered year-round library jobs and summer research stipends.

SOCIAL LIFE

The social life here is interspersed between exam periods. Groups regularly get together for golf, card games, dances, and other activities. The students at Marshall are generally older, and for the most part, "laid-back with some gunners."

COMMENTS: The best part about this school is its cost, which is reasonable for West Virginia residents and for nonresidents. The clinical facilities are either modern or are currently being renovated, and for the most part, they are adequate. Students find that the small class size gives them greater opportunities for individual attention and that both the faculty and administration are interested in their concerns.

MAYO MEDICAL SCHOOL
200 First Street, S.W.   /   Rochester, Minnesota 55905

LOCATION: Small City

AGE OF SCHOOL: 16 Years

CONTROL: Private (With state subsidy)

AMCAS **MEMBER:** Yes

CLASS SIZE: 40

PERCENT WOMEN IN CLASS: 50

PERCENT MINORITIES IN CLASS: 10

AVERAGE STUDENT EXPENDITURE: $$ (In-state); $$$ (Nonresident)

M.D.-Ph.D.:   Yes—biochemistry, cell biology, immunology, molecular biology, pathology, pharmacology, and physiology

NBME **Part I:** Students must record a score.

NBME **Part II:** Students must record a score.

PHYSICAL ENVIRONMENT

The medical complex at Mayo is eclectic, a mixture of old stone buildings and mirrored-glass structures. The Student Center is a recently renovated public library. The buildings are all within a few block radius (except for St. Mary's Hospital, which is a mile away) and are connected by underground passageways. Although Mayo has no campus per se, there is a YMCA four to five blocks away and a student lounge/gameroom. The school makes up for the lack of athletic facilities by sponsoring student teams to play in the town recreational leagues.

Mayo is famous for the Mayo Clinic, and the facilities at the school are excellent. The school is presently building another clinical building and a new education building. There is $50 million worth of construction in downtown Rochester associated with Mayo. The hospitals used most frequently by Mayo medical students are St. Mary's and Rochester Methodist Hospital. St. Mary's is a very large hospital and is often considered among the best in the nation. It is both old and new, with some areas over 90 years old and others recently renovated. A shuttle bus takes students from the clinic here to all other associated buildings. There is a large trauma center at this facility. Methodist Hospital is a newer hospital, about 15 years old, and is very well designed and efficient. It is one block north of the Mayo Clinic and downtown with all other clinical buildings. Very little time is spent by students doing "scut work" because of the efficiency of ancillary personnel and the lab/x-ray system.

Without question, the clinical facilities at Mayo are one of its strongest features, including the planned opening of regional group practices in the southeastern and southwestern United States. Students find that they are exposed to an incredibly large variety of SES patients, with health care delivery facilities ranging from rural clinics to the most state-of-the-art diagnostic facilities in a tertiary care medical center.

Rochester, Minnesota, is a small city often described as a "suburb without a city." The area around the school is very clean and safe.

It is easy to locate housing, although there is no on-campus housing for medical students. A single apartment runs about $300 per month. Shared houses and apartments are the most common form of housing. Having a car would be nice in this area, but it is not a necessity because of the shuttle buses and proximity to clinical facilities.

ACADEMICS

The course work is more comprehensive and there is more to learn in a shorter period of time than at undergraduate school. Students recommend speech or communications classes, microbiology, and biochemistry before beginning medical school. The recent change in grading, which added an Honors grade to the Pass/Marginal/Fail system has increased competition among students a little, but not nearly as much as had been expected.

Mayo's curriculum is innovative. Students learn the basic sciences by a body-system approach their first year, as well as how to perform histories and physicals in the course Introduction to the Patient. The second year furthers the students' hands-on experience with six-week clerkships under the supervision of physician preceptors. There are excellent opportunities for research during a "research semester" in the third year, when half the class participates in a 21-week research semester while the other half is in clinical clerkships. The fourth year is almost all electives but includes a six-week internal medicine clerkship required of all students.

Anatomy, pharmacology, and neuroscience are considered among the hardest courses faced by students at Mayo. Students advise studying in small groups to go over material and quiz one another. One man says, "Review the material until you understand it. Don't just memorize it!" The faculty is very good, and many of the first-year courses are taught by clinicians, which makes the material seem much more relevant.

FINANCIAL

Mayo is a private school; however, because of state subsidies, the cost for attending depends to a great extent on residency. Out-of-staters spend about $26,000 per year, while in-staters spend about $17,000 per year. The school has a loan program similar to GSL. Many students take out GSLs as well. There are some job opportunities at the school's medical center and library, and students can participate in medical research for a stipend.

SOCIAL LIFE

Mayo's advisor system—which breaks the class into groups of four students, a junior medical student, and a permanent faculty member—is designed to make certain that students have a smooth transition from college to medical school. There are many social functions organized by students and student organizations. The school sponsors one party and an evening called "Mixed Bag," which is a talent and skit-type show complete with chili supper and dancing afterward. There are also gatherings for each class during the year at the deans' homes or at one of the former Mayo mansions. The class is diverse, and about half of the 40 students are from out of state. Students here are impressed with Mayo's strong emphasis on patient care. The patient is always number one, and a humanitarian type of medicine is taught in a very high-tech environment.

COMMENTS: Overall, this is one of the best places to be for those interested in learning medicine with a great deal of individual attention and phenomenal clinical facilities (the Mayo Clinic is world-famous). This school has gone to great lengths to give its students outstanding clinical opportunities.

MEDICAL COLLEGE OF OHIO (TOLEDO)
C.S. No. 10008 / Toledo, Ohio 43699

LOCATION: Suburban/Big City

AGE OF SCHOOL: 24 Years

CONTROL: Public/State

AMCAS **MEMBER:** Yes

CLASS SIZE: 136

PERCENT WOMEN IN CLASS: 33

PERCENT MINORITIES IN CLASS: 12

AVERAGE STUDENT EXPENDITURE: $ (In-state); $$ (Nonresident)

M.D.-Ph.D.: No

NBME **Part I:** Students must record a score.

NBME **Part II:** Students must record a score.

PHYSICAL ENVIRONMENT

The medical school buildings, made of limestone, are modern and have many large windows. Two new buildings are under construction. This is an autonomous medical/graduate school; thus, the campus is the medical school. All facilities are compact and easily accessible. A new fitness center opened in 1986, and there is a recreation area located on the top floor of the Hospital Support Building, which is connected to the lecture hall building by tunnels. The classrooms are described as "luxurious."

The buildings and all the facilities are relatively new. Renovation is not a concern at this point, but construction of new facilities, redecoration, and updating of present technology is continual. The clinical facilities are excellent, and the school is currently building a new outpatient clinic building. The primary hospital facility is the

Medical College of Ohio Hospital, a very attractive and modern facility that is well staffed and administered. The school also has the Child and Adolescent Psychiatric Hospital and Comprehensive Rehabilitation Hospital on the campus, and there is the possibility of an NMR (Nuclear Magnetic Resonance) facility being built in the future. There are also plans to build a running track on the perimeter of the entire campus. Students feel that they are exposed to a wide variety of patients through the course of their rotations.

The school is set back in a wooded ravine with access from two main roads. It has two apartment complexes bounding it on its other sides. It is not difficult to locate inexpensive housing near the school. A one-bedroom apartment runs about $300 per month, while a three-bedroom townhouse is $395 per month. There are no dorms, so most students either share houses or live in apartments.

ACADEMICS

Students feel that there is much emphasis on learning details, many of which are unnecessary and not needed in clinical areas. It is recommended that premeds take only the minimum prerequisites before entering and take nonsciences instead in order to broaden their interests and experiences before medical school. Competition for grades does not get intense among most graduate students because grades are Pass/Fail and no ranking is posted. Anatomy was difficult for most students because of the level of minutia tested as well as the great emphasis placed on the course (one full year with cadaver).

Doing well at this school is based on effective time management. One woman says, "Every medical [student] has advice as to how to 'make it' in med school. No one system is better or worse than another. The incoming student would do best to examine which study methods have worked best for him [or her] in the past, then apply them to med school."

Most students do not have a lot of contact with faculty unless they are in academic trouble, although there are some exceptions. The clinical faculty, especially in internal medicine, are excellent. However, at times the clinical experiences in the last two years can be weakened by the low patient census at some of the affiliated hospitals. There are research opportunities during the summer between the first and second years and during clinical electives. Many students publish their research.

FINANCIAL

The cost of a year at the Medical College of Ohio runs about $15,000 for residents and $17,000 for nonresidents. There are many scholarships and grants, as well as low-interest loans, available to medical students. Medical College of Ohio has a college work/study program that allows 10 hours of work per week. These jobs are flexible and allow students to work around their school schedule.

SOCIAL LIFE

There are many opportunities for social interaction at this school, especially during the first two years. There is usually a social gathering every weekend, as well as a film club, about five dances per year, and the graduation party. The students are very easygoing, diversified, and friendly people who know how to combine studying with a social life.

COMMENTS: Students at the Medical College of Ohio (MCO) are enthusiastic about the enormous progress their school has made in such a short period of time. One woman says, "I think one of the strengths of MCO is its progressive curriculum in such areas as alcoholism, nutrition, and medical ethics. . . . The student affairs office is very good at trying to address the student's needs and act as student advocates." Another student adds, "MCO is a growing school and there is no way to escape this feeling while you are here. . . . The school is growing both in name and number. The new building will add much to the campus and a new dean is already laying out long-range academic and curriculum goals."

MEHARRY MEDICAL COLLEGE

1005 D.B. Todd Jr. Boulevard   /   Nashville, Tennessee 37208

LOCATION: Urban/Big City
AGE OF SCHOOL: 112 Years
CONTROL: Private
AMCAS MEMBER: No
SIZE OF CLASS: 80

PERCENT WOMEN IN CLASS: 45

PERCENT MINORITIES IN CLASS: 90

AVERAGE STUDENT EXPENDITURE: $$ (Both in-state and nonresident)

M.D.-Ph.D.: Yes—anatomy, biochemistry, microbiology, pharmacology, and through Division of Biological Sciences

NBME **Part I:** Passing score required for promotion

NBME **Part II:** Passing score required for graduation

PHYSICAL ENVIRONMENT

Meharry Medical College is housed in a modern building with good instructional facilities and spacious classrooms. The area around the school is considered somewhat safe if proper precautions are exercised at night. The school has excellent facilities, including The International Center for Health Sciences, which has the major function of coordinating internships and field study in order to help both African and United States health professionals assist in introducing maternal child health services to African countries. The library is spacious and has student study areas and computer bibliographic capabilities through the National Library of Medicine and through DIALOG information retrieval services. Athletic facilities are easily available for students.

George Russell Towers of Meharry/Hubbard Hospital is the major hospital out of which students rotate. This facility has modern equipment, a good nursing staff, and good opportunities for students to see a wide variety of patients and cases. The Community Mental Health Center (CMHC) serves a wide spectrum of patients, from children to senior citizens. There are also numerous VA hospital affiliations. Students are able to learn under the supervision of private practitioners across the country for family and community medicine.

Students find that it is not difficult to find reasonably priced housing in the area of the school, with the average one-bedroom apartment costing between $200 and $300 per month. Meharry has on-campus accommodations that includes Dorothy Brown Hall, which is open to female students and costs $121 per month for a double and $133 per month for a single room. The Student-Faculty Towers, which students say is a very nice apartment complex, costs from $175 to $255 per month.

ACADEMICS

Students strongly recommend having a sound background in the basic sciences before attending this medical school. Recommended courses include anatomy, microbiology, biochemistry, and the social sciences, particularly psychology ("They'll help you to relate to the patients"). Methods of studying that students find successful at Meharry are studying in groups, being very organized, and "putting as much time in as possible."

The faculty is regarded highly, and one student says, "They're there when you really need them. . . . The lectures are not repetitive or boring, but instead offer insight and understanding." There are numerous research opportunities that are showcased each year by a Student Research Day. Competition for grades is not intense ("It's best to compete against yourself and not your classmates"), although the school uses a letter grading system to evaluate students.

Meharry offers qualified students (in the top quartile of the applicant pool) a chance to enter the Medical Scholars Program, which begins the summer before the first year to give students special instruction in the biomedical sciences. These students have the option of participating in combined M.D.-Ph.D./M.D.-M.S. programs or the regular four-year program. The curriculum has recently introduced more electives and free time for students to pursue their individual interests. Clinical correlations are made by clinicians with the involvement of patients in order to enhance student understanding.

FINANCIAL

Meharry will cost first-year students an average of $16,000, regardless of residency. There are numerous loans and scholarships administered by the school, and many students take out federal loans, including GSL, NDSL, and HEAL. Although working is discouraged by both the administration and students ("It's too much of a drain for the small amount of money you'll get"), laboratory and medically related jobs are available for students.

SOCIAL LIFE

There are social activities for students, such as parties and student-faculty get-togethers. Meharry has a large number of fraternities and sororities, and there is an active chapter of AMSA on campus. Students here describe themselves as hardworking, self-motivated, and fun loving.

COMMENTS: Meharry has a strong medical program and offers several advantages, including good clinical facilities, a very strong faculty, many research opportunities, and an open and dedicated administration.

MERCER UNIVERSITY
School of Medicine
1550 College Street   /   Macon, Georgia 31207

LOCATION: Medium-Sized City

AGE OF SCHOOL: 6 Years

CONTROL: Private

AMCAS **MEMBER:**   Yes

CLASS SIZE: 24

PERCENT CLASS WOMEN: 38

PERCENT CLASS MINORITY: 13

AVERAGE STUDENT EXPENDITURE: $$ (Both in-state and nonresident)

M.D.-Ph.D.:   No

NBME **Part I:**   Passing score required for promotion

NBME **Part II:**   Passing score required for graduation

PHYSICAL ENVIRONMENT

Mercer University School of Medicine is housed in a new building in Macon, which is often called the "biggest little town in Georgia." The classroom facilities are exceptional. Students rotate primarily out of the Medical Center of Central Georgia. Students find this to be an adequate clinical facility, as is the school's ambulatory care unit.

The medical school has its own free gym, and there is a $7 fee for pool membership from May to October. It is very easy to find housing at many prices, ranging from $175 to $375 per month. Most students elect to live in apartments. The area around the school is considered relatively safe. Students find that having a car is a decided advantage at this school.

ACADEMICS

One of Mercer's primary missions is the training of physicians who will serve in rural and underserviced areas of Georgia. There are no courses; rather, learning is accomplished in "phases" using a multidisciplinary approach. These phases are far more challenging than undergraduate courses, so it is recommended that students take physiology, psychology, and embryology, and have a good background in human anatomy before attending Mercer. The first three phases comprise what is known as the Biochemical Problem Solving Unit and include such areas as communication occurring at various structural levels; the reaction of humans to their environment; the function and structure of disease (accomplished through means of a pathophysiological approach); clinical clerkships through the major specialties; the Community Service Program, which occurs in a rural setting in conjunction with the school's mission; and student electives.

Students do not find that there is much "open competition" at this school. The faculty here are excellent, and there are actually more faculty than students, which translates into outstanding opportunities for personal attention. Research opportunities are abundant, with five laboratories that are engaged in research and encourage and welcome student help.

FINANCIAL

Mercer costs a total of $20,000 for the first year, regardless of state residency. The school awards limited financial aid to students who demonstrate need. Most students take out federal loans. There are some jobs at this school, but the pay is not very good and students find that a job is not worth the amount of time that is taken away from studying and their lives outside medical school.

SOCIAL LIFE

There are only 24 students in each class, but there are a good number of social activities organized by students, including banquets, luncheons, seminars, parties, and intramural sports. The class is made up of "laid back and very personable people."

COMMENTS: Mercer is one of the youngest medical schools in the United States. It offers its students phenomenal opportunities for interaction with and attention from faculty and an innovative curriculum. As one student says, "I cannot imagine a more stress-free medical curriculum." Georgia residents are given preference for admissions. This is an oustanding school for those interested in practicing primary care medicine.

MICHIGAN STATE UNIVERSITY
College of Human Medicine
East Lansing, Michigan 48824

LOCATION: Big City

CONTROL: Public/State

AGE OF SCHOOL: 24 Years

AMCAS **MEMBER:**   Yes

SIZE OF CLASS: 106

PERCENT WOMEN IN CLASS: 50

PERCENT MINORITIES IN CLASS: 15

AVERAGE STUDENT EXPENDITURE: $ (In-state); $$ (Nonresidents)

M.D.-Ph.D.:   Yes—available in conjunction with numerous basic and behaviorial sciences

NBME **Part I:**   Passing score required for promotion

NBME **Part II:**   Passing score required for graduation

PHYSICAL ENVIRONMENT

Michigan State University College of Human Medicine is housed in a gray cement building that one student says "looks like a storage building." The rest of the Michigan State University (a Big Ten School) is beautiful, and the campus offers medical students fantastic resources, such as athletic and cultural facilities and restaurants. Inside, the lecture facilities are adequate.

Students begin their clinical instruction on campus in an ambulatory care facility. The third- and fourth-year rotations are conducted at community-based hospitals. Michigan State uses 17 community-based hospitals in 8 Michigan cities—including Lansing, Kalamazoo, and Grand Rapids—so the clinical sites are not on one campus. Michigan State has excellent and extensive clinical facilities, and students comment that they see a wide variety of patients from various backgrounds, with cases ranging from minor abrasions to complex medical problems.

The area surrounding the school is safe. The cost of an apartment is about $250 per month. Most students prefer this form of housing. As several students point out, "The atmosphere varies depending on which city you choose to fit your learning needs."

ACADEMICS

If the exterior of the instructional center of Michigan State is bland, the innovative curriculum being taught inside this building more than compensates for this fact. The curriculum is based on G. L. Engle's biopsychosocial model, so students planning on attending this school would benefit from reading his work. Students also recommend taking social sciences ("especially sociology and psychology"), anatomy, physiology, ethics, and biochemistry before attending. There is little competition for grades, which are Honors/Pass/Fail.

The curriculum is divided into three major phases that, like Engle's model, integrate biological, social, and clinical sciences, including a clinical segment in which students do rotations at the community hospital of their choosing. The first phase is only one semester and serves as an introduction to basic sciences, clinical skills, and medicine. The second phase is split into two tracks, and students can opt either for traditional instruction in basic sciences or for small-group problem-oriented learning, which entails greater freedom and thus the need for more self-motivation on the part of the student. The final phase involves choosing a community hospital associated with the college for clinical training.

The faculty at this school are considered excellent lecturers who are fully involved with and truly believe in the educational philosophies of Michigan State. There are opportunities for research, including M.D.-Ph.D. programs in both the basic sciences and humanities.

FINANCIAL

Michigan State University College of Human Medicine is a very good value for state residents. It costs about $13,500 for residents and $20,000 for nonresidents. The school has an excellent financial aid office, and several students take out loans. It is possible to work while enrolled here, especially the first two years, and the school will help find work for those who need it.

SOCIAL LIFE

Because of its location on the main campus (a school where 16,000 people live on campus and 40,000 attend classes) there are numerous opportunities for socializing outside the classroom. There are school-planned parties and gatherings. The class is diverse, and students here describe themselves as "mainly humanistic folks."

COMMENTS: You may notice that the name of this school is somewhat unusual—Michigan State University College of Human Medicine. It is not just the name that is different. The curriculum is innovative and progressive, and the approach to clinical training is rather unusual and, by most student accounts, highly effective. Michigan State is an excellent school to consider if you are interested in attending a school that is not overly competitive and has good facilities and an outstanding faculty and student body.

MOREHOUSE SCHOOL OF MEDICINE
830 Westview Drive, S.W.   /   Atlanta, Georgia 30314

LOCATION: Urban

AGE OF SCHOOL: 10 Years

CONTROL: Private

AMCAS **MEMBER:** Yes

CLASS SIZE: 32

PERCENT OF WOMEN IN CLASS: 41

PERCENT OF MINORITIES IN CLASS: 85

AVERAGE STUDENT EXPENDITURE: $$ (Both in-state and nonresident)

M.D.-Ph.D.: No

NBME **Part I:** Passing score required for promotion

NBME **Part II:** Passing score required for graduation

PHYSICAL ENVIRONMENT

Morehouse School of Medicine is in a new building that is less than five years old. A new clinical sciences building is almost finished. Both buildings are modern and well kept. The school's library is small but excellent, and the laboratory facilities are adequate. The facilities for teaching physical diagnosis are currently in need of work. However, there is planned renovation of these facilities. Morehouse is surrounded by other black institutions, including Spellman College, Clark College, Morris Brown College, and Atlanta University.

Morehouse has a broad range of hospital affiliations that provide students with the chance to observe a wide spectrum of both patients (ranging from very low SES to high SES) and cases. Grady Hospital (shared with Emory) is the major clinical site and generally serves a lower SES patient. This facility provides excellent exposure to complex and simple medical problems. Southwest Community Hospital houses a Family Practice Residency in which students treat patients from primarily middle and upper SES backgrounds.

A gym and other campus facilities are close by and available for students. The school is immediately surrounded by low-income housing in what is considered a relatively safe area. It is not difficult to locate suitable housing; however, most apartment complexes are from 5 to 20 miles from the school. Most students live in apartments, and the average cost for a one-bedroom apartment is between $200 and $300 per month.

ACADEMICS

Students find the work to be far more demanding than what they were accustomed to as undergraduates. One student recommends that prospective students "take courses which stress the ability to articulate ideas and communicate with others. They'll teach you what you need at med school. Stress humanities, philosophy, reading, and writing." Students are conscious of their grades but not obsessed with them, and competition is discouraged (grading system: A/B/C/D/F and P/F.)

Gross anatomy, pathology, and physiology are considered to be among the most challenging basic sciences. It is recommended that students seek help as soon as they run into difficulty with the material, for "procastination is your own worst enemy." Self-testing and reviewing by integrating small facts into broader concepts are also considered good study methods.

The faculty are considered good, with a few teachers who "enjoy building up an adversarial relationship with students." By and large, students think very highly of the faculty and comment that the small class size makes it possible for the faculty to know students individually. There are adequate research opportunities at this school.

FINANCIAL

The first year at Morehouse will cost a total of approximately $20,000, regardless of residency. Morehouse has its own loan/scholarship program, and many students take out federal loans. One student says that "financial aid at this school is a real puzzle. Nobody has been able to fathom their methodology [for awarding aid]." Students feel that it is possible to work about 10 hours a week through Morehouse's work/study program.

SOCIAL LIFE

There are several social events for students, including a talent show, parties, and picnics. Students at this school have strong personalities and viewpoints. The area around the school offers numerous cultural and entertainment possibilities through participation in the activities of the neighboring colleges.

COMMENTS: Morehouse has the major advantage of a small class, which gives students a great deal of individual attention. One woman adds, "It is a very good institution. It is constantly learning and revising and is destined to be one of the bigger medical schools in the future."

MOUNT SINAI SCHOOL OF MEDICINE
City University of New York
One Gustave L. Levy Place   /   New York, New York 10029

LOCATION: Big City/Urban

AGE OF SCHOOL: 25 Years

CONTROL: Private

AMCAS **MEMBER:** No

CLASS SIZE: 115

PERCENT WOMEN IN CLASS: 45

PERCENT MINORITIES IN CLASS: 6

AVERAGE STUDENT EXPENDITURE: $$$$ (Both in-state and nonresident)

M.D.-Ph.D.: Yes—anatomy, biochemistry, pathology, genetics, microbiology, neurobiology, pharmacology, and physiology; also, The Fifth Pathway, a program available to students who went to U.S. colleges, were unable to get into U.S. medical schools, and attended foreign medical schools. This program is designed to help students refine their clinical skills before seeking internships/residencies in the United States.

NBME **Part I:** Passing score required for promotion

NBME **Part II:** Passing score required for graduation

PHYSICAL ENVIRONMENT

Mount Sinai School of Medicine is across the street from Central Park, which most students enjoy during the daytime. The building for the first- and second-year classes is the Annenberg Building, which is beautiful, modern, and clean. Mount Sinai Hospital itself is a very old building that is presently being renovated "one pavilion at a time." Most in-patient floors are located in antiquated buildings. However, a new in-patient hospital complex is under construction.

Students feel that facilities do not keep pace with the high-technology equipment available to them. One student comments, "It makes for an interesting juxtaposition, [the advanced technology equipment] against a physical plant which was built decades ago." But, as stated earlier, the plant is slowly being rebuilt to accomodate the new and sophisticated equipment.

The clinical years are spent at Mount Sinai Hospital; Elmhurst (Queens) Hospital, which is a city hospital; Beth Israel Medical Center, a modern, well-run facility; and the Bronx VA hospital, which is a new facility.

Mount Sinai is near Spanish Harlem, which is not the safest area to walk alone in at night. But students claim that reports of a high neighborhood crime rate are exaggerated. Mount Sinai is not affiliated with an undergraduate campus, but there is a small weight room in the dormitory, as well as free passes to a nearby YMCA. Students have access to Hunter High School gym for intramural sports.

The school is in the heart of Manhattan and Mount Sinai provides housing at less than market values. Buyer beware. The cost of housing around the school is still expensive, although most students say that they find themselves very fortunate to be living in the school's housing. Student housing averages $600 per month, which would cost about $1200 per month on the open market. There are dorm rooms for single students; married students generally live in apartments.

ACADEMICS

The difficulty of courses at Mount Sinai arises from the tremendous amount of memorization. The work is not conceptually difficult, and most courses organize the material for you, which makes it easier to "consume the information." Biochemistry is highly recommended, but one student feels there are no courses necessary other than the traditional premed sciences. He encourages students to take whatever they want during their undergraduate years.

Tests are graded fairly. Competition for grades is not intense in the first two years, when evaluations are Pass/Fail. The third year is slightly more competitive, although not too terrible, because students are still willing to help one another when "push comes to shove." Medicine and pediatrics are among the hardest courses because there's a great deal to know and not a lot of time to master all the material.

The key to success at this school (and at any school for that matter) is discipline. You need to stick to your schedule over the "long haul." You cannot be haphazard about your studying.

FINANCIAL

Mount Sinai is an expensive medical school to attend because it is a private school and because it is located in one of the costliest cities in the nation (if not the world). Depending on living accommodations and style of living, Mount Sinai will cost a single student between $25,000 and $30,000 per year total. The school provides occasional job opportunities but does not encourage students to work during the year. It is more possible to work during the first two years than during the last two years. Most students get partial financial aid through a combination of loans and some grants.

SOCIAL LIFE

There are a fair number of social events, including the first-year class play and weekend parties. Manhattan has more cultural offerings than any person could take advantage of in a lifetime including ballet, opera, and museums. Students at Mount Sinai are a driven bunch, many of whom are native New Yorkers. They comment about the well-roundedness of their school's curriculum and the school's willingness to help students.

COMMENTS: Mount Sinai is working toward the improvement of an already fine medical school with a friendly and highly competent student body. The school has an outstanding faculty and very fine clinical facilities.

NEW YORK MEDICAL COLLEGE

Elmwood Hall   /   Valhalla, New York 10595

LOCATION: Suburban/Medium-Sized City

AGE OF SCHOOL: 128 Years

CONTROL: Private

AMCAS **MEMBER:** Yes

SIZE OF CLASS: 186

PERCENT WOMEN IN CLASS: 40

PERCENT MINORITIES IN CLASS: 15

AVERAGE STUDENT EXPENDITURE: $$$$$ (Both in-state and nonresident)

M.D.-Ph.D.: Yes—anatomy, biochemistry, microbiology, pathology, pharmacology and physiology; also, combined M.D.-Masters of Public Health (M.P.H.) available

NBME **Part I:** Students must record a score.

NBME **Part II:** Students must record a score.

PHYSICAL ENVIRONMENT

New York Medical College is located in Valhalla, which is a suburban part of Westchester County. The school is housed in an attractive facility aptly named the Basic Sciences Building. The classroom and laboratory facilities are considered very up to date and modern, "particularly the anatomy lab." There is a basketball court on campus, and there are nearby athletic and recreational facilities for tennis, hockey, skating, softball, and football. The area surrounding the school is relatively safe.

The strongest feature of New York Medical School is its numerous clinical affiliations with a total of more than 14,000 beds. New York Medical has affiliates in a variety of suburban and urban locations, including St. Vincent's Hospital and Medical Center in New York City, an outstanding facility; Harlem Valley Psychiatric Center; Kingston Hospital; Yonkers General Hospital; St. Francis Hospital (both Poughkeepsie and Roslyn); New York Eye and Ear Infirmary; Montrose VA Hospital; and numerous other clinical facilities. Few other medical schools offer students the opportunity to rotate out of and study at such a wide variety of health care facilities. There is no question (as is confirmed by students) that students are exposed to an enormous spectrum of patients ranging from the lowest to highest SES and a greater diversity of cases of all complexities.

Finding housing near the school poses a mild problem, but the housing office is somewhat helpful in locating rooms and apartments for students. The average cost for a one-bedroom apartment is between $300 and $400 per month. It is recommended that students bring a car to get around Westchester, although the bus system is good.

ACADEMICS

"Take the fun courses while you still have the time. But don't just take the basic premed requirements, add on a few advanced courses like biochemistry and human anatomy. It'll make your first year a lot easier." Students do not find their classmates to be cutthroat or overtly competitive (Pass/Fail for basic sciences). The first year consists primarily of basic sciences and an interesting course entitled Behavioral Science that holds lectures about such topics as patient-doctor relationships, statistics and research techniques, and an introduction to disordered behavior. The introduction to clinical medicine begins during the second year in a course with the same name. Third year is mostly clinical clerkships and rotations, and fourth year entails three months of required rotations and electives.

The faculty are "both research oriented and committed to teaching. A rare combination to find these days." Students speak very highly of their instructors and add that there are numerous opportunities for student research. Students recommend going over notes, attending all lectures, and being organized for optimal performance on exams.

FINANCIAL

Perhaps the biggest complaint about New York Medical School is its very high cost. The first year will cost a total of $32,000, regardless of state residency. There are numerous financial aid programs recommended by the school and students, including GSL, ALAS, HEAL, NDSL, and the Federal Health Professions Loan (HPL). New York State residents may qualify for the Tuition Assistance Program (TAP) if their family's net income is below $20,000 per year. Regents Scholarships are awarded to New York State residents who meet academic qualifications and also agree to practice in underserved areas in New York State.

SOCIAL LIFE

New York Medical students are involved in many activities, including a new student publication called *Progress*, an active chapter of AMSA, the annual production of "Follies," and a Student Physician Awareness Day. The students at this school are diversified and come from a wide variety of colleges and universities.

COMMENTS: No, this is not NYU Medical, which many people confuse the school with. New York Medical College has the distinct advantage of phenomenal clinical sites, a very strong faculty, and a good location. The very high cost of attending is a problem for students, but students find that they are able to make do by taking out several loans. The school has an excellent summer program for minority students.

NEW YORK UNIVERSITY
School of Medicine
550 First Avenue   /   New York, New York 10016

LOCATION: Urban/Big City

AGE OF SCHOOL: 147 Years

CONTROL: Private

AMCAS **MEMBER:** No

CLASS SIZE: 150

PERCENT WOMEN IN CLASS: 33

PERCENT MINORITIES IN CLASS: 2

AVERAGE STUDENT EXPENDITURE: $$$ (Both in-state and nonresident)

M.D.-Ph.D.: Yes—available in numerous basic sciences as well as social sciences

NBME **Part I:** Optional

NBME **Part II:** Optional

PHYSICAL ENVIRONMENT

Walking into the New York University (NYU) Medical Science Building, where first- and second-year students take their basic sciences, one is reminded of the history of medicine and the many advances that have come about since the horse-drawn ambulance housed in the lobby of this building was used. There are a series of underground tunnels that connect the medical school buildings; making it easier in bad weather for students to get to classes.

The school itself is located in a good section of New York and is accessible to the undergraduate campus by shuttle bus, subways, or even walking (about a mile away). Medical students are able to use athletic facilities on the Washington Square campus after paying a small fee, and there is a gym in Rubin Hall for a $10 membership fee, as well as numerous health clubs near the school. Safety is reasonable around the area of the school provided that students take precautions when walking at night.

Perhaps one of NYU's most attractive features is its clinical facilities, including the University Hospital, which has private patients and excellent ancillary personnel; New York Veterans Hospital, which houses older patients; and Bellevue Hospital which students find the most interesting of the three hospitals. Bellevue has a wide spectrum of SES patients and cases. According to one student, "The opportunities for seeing unique cases in medicine are staggering at this facility."

NYU medical students are fortunate in regard to housing because on-campus living is reasonably priced when compared to New York City rents and students can live in the dorms for all four years if they choose. The cost for a dorm room in Rubin Hall is between $200 and $300 per month. Sharing an apartment in Kips Bay Dorm, which is a preferable accommodation, costs about $375 per month.

ACADEMICS

Competing with their classmates for good grades is not a concern for students at this school. The grading policy is Pass/Fail, and students here are not ranked. There are numerous opportunities for student research, including the Honors Program, in which students conduct research under the supervision of a senior faculty member and write and defend a 20-page thesis for graduation with the medical degree with honors. M.D.-Ph.D. students, affectionately called "mudd phudds," are funded for the full six years of study (if they need an extra year, NYU picks up the cost) and are able to conduct research in either the basic or social sciences.

Students have experience with patients during their first year if they take the elective Clinical Correlations, which is under the supervision of a fourth-year medical student the first semester and an attending physician the second semester. The behavioral science course also gives students experience with both patients and the hospital sites.

The faculty here are considered among the top in their respective fields and accessible to students. The Student Life Committee involves students, faculty members, and administrators and gives students the opportunity to voice student concerns and change academic policies if needed.

As mentioned earlier, students are eager to learn but find that there is less pressure because of the grading system. The student-run note service is very well organized and helpful when it comes time to prepare for exams. It is recommended that premeds take as many humanities as possible while in college, as well as biochemistry. Physiology is considered to be among the most challenging, as well as one of the best-taught, courses at the school.

FINANCIAL

NYU School of Medicine will cost the average single student between $22,000 and $25,000 for the first year. The financial aid department is very helpful, and most students have taken out a loan of some sort. Though it is not recommended that students work their third year, there are several job opportunities in the hospital. Student researchers make about $175 per week during the summer (between 8 and 12 weeks).

SOCIAL LIFE

NYU medical students are both highly motivated and fun-loving. The class is diverse in backgrounds and interests but homogenous in geographic distribution (primarily from New York and New Jersey). The Student Affairs Office goes out of its way to organize as many social activities for students as possible, including providing reduced-price tickets to Broadway shows and area nightclubs and organizing parties. There are also Liver Rounds, which are parties sponsored by the upperclassmen. As far as outside cultural offerings, NYU is located a subway or bus ride away from anything possible outside the realm of school.

COMMENTS: If you are interested in advancing medicine and attending a school which is actively involved in research and has strong clinical instruction (particularly at Bellevue), then NYU may definitely be the place for you. The school attracts "the best and the brightest" students, who are highly motivated but are not "cutthroat" competitive. This medical school combines the "traditional" basic sciences approach with numerous opportunities for experience with patients early in your medical education.

NORTHWESTERN UNIVERSITY
Medical School
Ward Building 4-142
303 East Chicago Avenue / Chicago, Illinois 60611

LOCATION: Urban/Big City

AGE OF SCHOOL: 129 Years

CONTROL: Private (With state support)

AMCAS **MEMBER:** Yes

SIZE OF CLASS: 163

PERCENT WOMEN IN CLASS: 40

PERCENT MINORITIES IN CLASS: 5

AVERAGE STUDENT EXPENDITURE: $$$$ (Both in-state and nonresident)

M.D.-Ph.D.: Yes—anatomy, biochemistry, cell biology, clinical physiology, microbiology, immunology, molecular biology, neuroscience, pathology, pharmacology, physiology, and tumor biology; also; M.D.-Masters of Management (M.M.) with Kellog Graduate School of Management and M.D.-Masters of Public Health (M.P.H.) available, as well as a 7-year biomedical program with the undergraduate school

NBME **Part I:** Students must record a score.

NBME **Part II:** Optional

PHYSICAL ENVIRONMENT

In a time when many schools are cutting back on their budgets and building, Northwestern University Medical School is not only renovating current facilities but is also planning the construction of a 15-story facility for faculty research and student laboratories. Students find that the school makes every effort to accommodate their needs with regard to study facilities, including computer learning programs. The medical complex is about a 10-minute drive from the undergraduate Evanston campus, where there are numerous athletic facilities students can use.

Northwestern has a large number of clinical facilities for its students to rotate out of, including the McGraw Medical Center, made up of Evanston Hospital ("very modern facilities, equipment, and a good variety of patients"), Children's Memorial Hospital ("the site of heart transplants in children"), Northwestern Memorial Hospital ("excellent facility for critical care"), the Rehabilitation Institute of Chicago ("treats a variety of patients with problems such as strokes, multiple sclerosis, and also has a great physical therapy department"), and Lakeside VA hospital. Students find that through these facilities and other affiliated clinical facilities, they see a very wide spectrum of patients and cases.

The medical school is located in one of the nicest (as well as costliest) areas of Chicago and is considered safe for all practical purposes. Students strongly recommend the dormitories as a reasonably priced living accommodation that costs approximately $4200 including room and board (cafeteria in dorm). It is difficult to locate inexpensive off-campus housing, and the cost for a studio is close to $5000 for the entire year.

ACADEMICS

The first year is primarily devoted to basic sciences instruction but also includes courses involving patients, such as Introduction to Clinical Medicine (required), Patient Perspectives electives, and clinical preceptorships. The second year gives students more free time for clinical experiences and continues the study of basic sciences. The remaining two years consist of clinical clerkships.

Competition is discouraged at this school, although students feel that "a little competition is healthy as long it doesn't get out of hand." Grades are Honors/Pass/Fail. The faculty are considered excellent, and there are numerous opportunities for student research. Students strongly recommend having a solid foundation in both basic sciences ("Take biochemistry. It'll help you in the long run") and the social sciences.

As far as study methods, students feel that it is unfair to students to recommend one method over another because the first year is a time when students should find what method works best for them. They do, however, stress good organizational skills, obtaining old tests whenever possible, and budgeting time efficiently.

FINANCIAL

Northwestern will cost first-year students a total of approximately $30,000, regardless of state residency. Most students take out a large combination of loans, including NDSL and HEAL. There are some work opportunities, such as working as an anatomy teaching assistant, but students advise against working, particularly during the first year ('It's a period of adjusting").

SOCIAL LIFE

Northwestern is situated in a very good area and there are limitless cultural and entertainment (such as jazz bars) opportunities near the medical school. Students say that they have time for outside interests, and there are parties sponsored by both the school and individual students.

COMMENTS: Northwestern Medical School has several advantages, including a great location, excellent clinical and laboratory facilities, an understanding and well-known faculty, and good research opportunities. The cost for attending this school is high, but students say it is possible to get by with a combination of loans.

OHIO STATE UNIVERSITY
College of Medicine
370 West Ninth Avenue / Columbus, Ohio 43210

LOCATION: Big City
AGE OF SCHOOL: 74

CONTROL: Public/State

AMCAS **MEMBER:** Yes

CLASS SIZE: 233

PERCENT WOMEN IN CLASS: 33

PERCENT MINORITIES IN CLASS: 5

AVERAGE STUDENT EXPENDITURE: $ (In-state); $$ (Nonresident)

M.D.-Ph.D.: Yes—available in conjunction with several basic sciences

NBME **Part I:** Lecture/Discussion Program (LDP) students must record a score. Independent Study Program (ISP) students must record a passing score for promotion.

NBME **Part II:** Passing score required for graduation

PHYSICAL ENVIRONMENT

The medical school is fairly modern (built in 1969) and large. The grounds are well kept and the undergraduate campus is very accessible. The College of Medicine is on the corner of campus and is therefore close enough to athletic buildings but adds one student, "not far enough away from undergraduates." There is also a brand-new health and physical recreation center for both faculty and students.

The basic sciences instructional facilities are excellent. The school is also renovating the older research labs and building a new Cancer Research Center. Ohio State has the benefit of a large number of outstanding hospital affiliates. The University Hospital is a well-staffed and well-administered facility. There are numerous affiliations with hospitals throughout Columbus, and there is also a very good mental retardation center.

The campus is surrounded by a suburban area. There are a shopping center to the west and apartment complexes to the west and east. A middle SES neighborhood is to the south of the school, and to the north is a low to middle SES neighborhood. There are many reasonably priced modern apartments in the immediate area of the school. Most students live within two miles of the school. The average rent, including utilities, is $240 per month for a one-bedroom apartment, $410 per month for a two-bedroom apartment, and $600 per month for a three-bedroom apartment. The apartments are more expensive the closer you are to the school.

ACADEMICS

Students strongly recommend taking biochemistry before attending this school, as well as physiology, microbiology, histology, and psychology. The school employs a Pass/Fail grading system, and students find that the level of competition is rather low. The first two years are primarily basic sciences and courses that introduce students to the clinical aspect of medicine. The remaining two years are occupied by clinical clerkships and nine months of electives and selectives during the final year of study.

The faculty are spoken well of although students find that there are large differences in the quality of teaching from department to department. Overall, the faculty are easily accessible and are willing to talk with students after classes. Research opportunities are plentiful, and there are also many student grants that are not difficult to obtain.

FINANCIAL

Ohio State will cost a total of $11,000 for residents and $19,000 for nonresidents. There are several loans administered by the school, and most students are on financial aid of some sort, with GSLs being very popular. There are opportunities for student employment, and students find it is possible to work while enrolled at this school.

SOCIAL LIFE

Ohio State University College of Medicine is situated very close to a large university that offers outstanding opportunities for social interaction, culture, and entertainment. Students find that there is time for socializing outside the classroom, and there are several parties and intramural sports for students. The vast majority of students are Ohio residents, and students describe their class as "hardworking, fun-loving, and very caring."

COMMENTS: Students selected this school based on its national reputation, excellent facilities, and its very reasonable cost for Ohio residents. Ohio State College of Medicine is an excellent medical school with numerous research opportunities for students. It is working harder to attract more qualified minority applicants.

ORAL ROBERTS UNIVERSITY
School of Medicine
7777 South Lewis Avenue / Tulsa, Oklahoma 74171

LOCATION: Suburban

AGE OF SCHOOL: 10 Years

CONTROL: Private (Religious affiliation: Evangelical Christianity)

AMCAS **MEMBER:** Yes

CLASS SIZE: 48

PERCENT WOMEN IN CLASS: 30

PERCENT MINORITIES IN CLASS: 10

AVERAGE STUDENT EXPENDITURE: $$$ (Both in-state and nonresident)

M.D.-Ph.D.: No

NBME **Part I:** Passing score required for promotion

NBME **Part II:** Passing score required for graduation

PHYSICAL ENVIRONMENT

Oral Roberts University School of Medicine was built a little more than eight years ago. It is a well-kept campus with very modern buildings. The school has excellent lecture and lab facilities and an adequate library. The City of Faith Medical and Research Center is the major teaching hospital, and students are exposed to both high and lower SES patients at this facility. The Colmery-O'Neil VA hospital is a large facility in very good condition. The Claremont Indian Hospital gives students a great deal of autonomy and is very popular among students.

Oral Roberts medical school is across the street from the main campus, which has athletic facilities such as an aerobics center with gym, a pool, a track, and racquetball courts. The school is located near one of the wealthiest residential areas ("The houses are so big they look like shopping centers") in Tulsa, which is very safe.

Locating housing does not pose a problem. According to one student, "Tulsa is in economic straits so everyone is selling or renting out their home." The school provides graduate housing ("well-furnished apartments about a quarter mile from campus") for single students and married students without children, which costs about

$300 per month for a two-bedroom apartment. Most students live in apartments.

ACADEMICS

"There is a greater amount of material to be mastered than in under-graduate science courses during the first two years here." Students recommend taking physiology, biochemistry, embryology, and humanities because "these can help you in unpredictable ways, such as understanding people of different backgrounds." A "healthy competition" for grades exists among students at Oral Roberts.

Repetition, reading as much of the required texts as possible, and integrating material are seen as keys to academic success at Oral Roberts. The faculty are described as "The best!" Several faculty invite students to their homes, and students feel that the faculty are truly concerned with the medical students' well-being.

Research opportunities are present, but "they do not come out and grab you." Students selected Oral Roberts for a variety of reasons, including its Christian emphasis, ability for overseas missions, its belief in whole-person medicine, the supportive faculty, and its outstanding student body.

FINANCIAL

Oral Roberts costs a total of about $21,000 for first-year students, regardless of state residency. Oral Roberts recently began its own loan program, which students find to be beneficial. Students also take out a combination of other loans, and there are some scholarships available. Although students feel it is not possible for students to work while enrolled at Oral Roberts, there are jobs for students' spouses.

SOCIAL LIFE

Oral Roberts students say that they are very close to their classmates. There are numerous social activities including Bible study and discussion groups. Students should be aware of the strong Christian philosophy of this school before considering applying here.

COMMENTS: Oral Roberts students are very proud of their school's accomplishments, such as recently receiving three-year (as opposed to one-year) accreditation. One student says, "Due to the fact that it [Oral Roberts] is trying to gain credibility in the medical community, they expect a little more from the students academically."

ROBERT WOOD JOHNSON MEDICAL SCHOOL

University of Medicine and Dentistry of New Jersey
P.O. Box 101 / Piscataway, New Jersey 08854

LOCATION: Suburban/Medium-Sized City

AGE OF SCHOOL: 22 Years

CONTROL: Public/State

AMCAS **MEMBER:** Yes

CLASS SIZE: 130

PERCENT WOMEN IN CLASS: 42

PERCENT MINORITIES IN CLASS: 10

AVERAGE STUDENT EXPENDITURE: $ (In-state); $$ (Nonresident)

M.D.-Ph.D.: Yes—available in conjunction with a wide variety of basic sciences

NBME **Part I:** Passing score required for promotion

NBME **Part II:** Passing score required for graduation

PHYSICAL ENVIRONMENT

Robert Wood Johnson Medical School is in a fairly modern structure. The research tower is attached to the teaching facilities, which gives students convenient access to professors' offices. The buildings are early-1970s cement-type architecture. The school is young and therefore all facilities are relatively new. A large construction job is about to begin on another research facility. First-year students are provided with microscopes, dissection kits, and lab coats without charge.

There are several hospital sites, including the University Hospital which has undergone extensive renovation at a cost of over $47 million. The French Street Development has an ambulatory surgery center; a cardiovascular institute; a bone, joint, and connective tissue institute; and state-of-the-art equipment. Robert Wood Johnson Medical School exposes its students to a wide variety of patients and cases.

There are numerous Rutgers University gyms open to medical students. Some are closer than others, but free campus buses take students to any or all of them. Many medical students work out, do aerobics, and play sports in these gyms. These facilities are quite good.

The school is located near a number of shopping areas. There are three large malls all within 10 to 20 minutes of the school. The school is only 50 minutes from Manhattan and 1½ hours from Philadelphia. It is in a very safe area, and there are no problems at night.

It is very easy to find housing. The school has organized dates in the summer for finding housing and always has lists of available locations. A two-bedroom apartment ranges from $250 to $450 per month for "nice" apartments. Most students live in apartments.

ACADEMICS

Students strongly recommend taking biochemistry, having a good familiarity with human anatomy, and pursuing interests in the humanities and the social sciences. The exams for the basic sciences are all multiple-choice. Students find that it can be quite competitive during the first year with the Honors/High Pass/Pass/Low Pass/ Fail grading system.

One student says about study methods, "Never fall behind in anatomy. Histology can be learned two weeks before an exam with no problem. Always understand what is being lectured on and dissected in anatomy beforehand. Otherwise, the time spent in class is useless."

The faculty at this school are considered outstanding and very accessible to students. "Some even attend our happy hours on Fridays." There are research opportunities over the summer that provide a stipend.

FINANCIAL

Robert Wood Johnson Medical School will cost about $17,000 for residents and $18,000 for nonresidents. Most students take out loans and strongly advise against working while at this school.

SOCIAL LIFE

Students are quite social, and there are happy hours every Friday night, as well as dinners and dances. Although some students in the classes are competitive, there is a sense of unity among students at this school.

COMMENTS: This school has an excellent faculty, very good clinical facilities, and a highly intelligent and gregarious student body.

ST. LOUIS UNIVERSITY
School of Medicine
1402 South Grand Boulevard   /   Saint Louis, Missouri 63104

LOCATION: Big City

AGE OF SCHOOL: 152 Years

CONTROL: Private (Religious affiliation: Jesuit)

AMCAS **MEMBER:** Yes

CLASS SIZE: 157

PERCENT WOMEN IN CLASS: 25

PERCENT MINORITIES IN CLASS: 2

AVERAGE STUDENT EXPENDITURE: $$$ (Both in-state and nonresident)

M.D.-Ph.D.: Yes—anatomy, biochemistry, microbiology, pathology, pharmacology, physiology, and virology

NBME **Part I:** Passing grade required for promotion

NBME **Part II:** Passing grade required for graduation

PHYSICAL ENVIRONMENT

St. Louis University School of Medicine is the first medical school organized west of the Mississippi River. The original buildings are old, but the buildings have been well kept and appropriately renovated. The Learning Resource Center is fairly new. The medical school itself is a conglomerate of four buildings. The newest addition is the animal care unit.

The Medical Center is also partly old, but the new Bordley Pavilion, scheduled for completion in 1987, houses all patient beds and research space. The old hospital will be renovated for office space and labs. There are many hospital sites for students, including the University Hospital, which has an academic atmosphere and good ancillary services. There are a lot of indigent patients here, so it makes up for a city/county hospital affiliation. Cardinal Glennon Memorial Hospital for Children is next to the University Hospital and is connected. This is a reasonably good facility with a strong pediatric program. The VA Hospital has a new addition, and students do a lot more "scut work" here. There is a great deal of autonomy here, especially in the surgery rotation. Jefferson Barracks is where students often go for psychiatry and medicine rotations. There are three private hospitals, the Deaconess Hospital, St.Mary's Health Center, and St. John's, all of which give limited autonomy to students.

North Campus, which is also Frost Campus as well as the undergraduate campus, is less than a mile away from the medical school and University Medical Center. There is also a bus system, The Fireline, that runs between the two campuses. There is a graduate dormitory. One very big highlight of the physical environment of St. Louis University is the Recreation Center which is much like a health club to which every medical student automatically belongs. The medical students are the largest user group of the facilities, which include an indoor track, a pool, weight rooms, racquetball courts, and multipurpose courts. There are many intramural sports that medical students participate in as well.

The area surrounding the school is described as a "ghetto." However,there's a big rehabilitation effort to improve things. The area is not considered very safe to walk in at night. Housing is easy to find, with first-year students having the option of living in dormitory rooms. A three-bedroom apartment costs about $350 to $375 per month.

ACADEMICS

The volume of material covered in a day is the equivalent of one week of undergraduate work. Students recommend statistics, ethics, biochemistry, and business and humanities courses before entering. There is not much competition for grades, especially with the

Pass/Fail grading option. Surprisingly, there are still a few "gunners" in each class. The hardest courses are systemic pathology, introduction to medicine, biochemistry, and physiology. Organization, such as putting each disease studied into a category, is the key for doing well in courses. Develop quality rather than quantity study habits because the amount of information is so great it is better to master less than to not understand a greater amount.

The faculty are very accessible, and many seem very willing to help in whatever way possible. There are opportunities for research during elective times, and there are summer grant opportunities that including NIH (National Institute of Health) positions.

FINANCIAL

The total for a year at St. Louis medical school is about $25,000, regardless of state residency. There are many free shows in St. Louis, which helps keep social costs down. About 70 to 80 percent of students have loans. Working is prohibited by the school and is grounds for disciplinary action and possible expulsion. The philosophy is that your first job is to learn and then you will be gainfully employed and able to readily repay loans.

SOCIAL LIFE

There is much opportunity for social life here, with extensive sports teams, talent shows, get-togethers (TGIF parties every other Friday with free beer, wine, and snacks), Christmas and Halloween parties, and a formal each spring. Collectively the class has experienced and helped each other through many ups and downs. St. Louis Medical School attracts diversified students from across the country.

COMMENTS: St. Louis School of Medicine offers very good clinical facilities, a fine faculty, and excellent opportunities for research.

SOUTHERN ILLINOIS UNIVERSITY
School of Medicine
P.O. Box 3926 / Springfield, Illinois 62708

LOCATION: Small Town

AGE OF SCHOOL: 19 Years

CONTROL: Public/State

AMCAS **MEMBER:** Yes

CLASS SIZE: 72

PERCENT WOMEN IN CLASS: 33

PERCENT MINORITIES IN CLASS: 5

AVERAGE STUDENT EXPENDITURE: $ (Generally, there are no out-of-state students in attendance.)

M.D.-Ph.D.: No

NBME **Part I:** Optional

NBME **Part II:** Optional

PHYSICAL ENVIRONMENT

Southern Illinois University School of Medicine is divided into two campuses. The first year is spent in Carbondale, Illinois, where the medical school is housed in a functional rectangular building located in a fairly safe area. The remaining three years are spent at Springfield, Illinois, in a spacious facility with an enclosed courtyard, extensive laboratory facilities, and a beautiful library.

Carbondale is "on-campus" and has a brand-new recreation center. Springfield has no "real" campus but is located across the street from a major tertiary care hospital. There are computers available for students in Springfield. The clinical sites are considered "more than adequate," and students find that by rotating through Memorial Medical Center and St. John's Hospital, both located in Springfield, they are exposed to a good variety of patients and cases.

Finding housing in either Carbondale or Springfield is no problem. Carbondale is described by one student as "the pits" and, ironically, has a higher cost of housing, with a single-bedroom apartment costing about $300 per month. Springfield is a "big small town" and has a wide variety of housing, averaging about $250 per month for a one-bedroom apartment. Most students share either apartments or houses in both locations.

ACADEMICS

Southern Illinois has an innovative curriculum, with courses taught by an organ-system approach rather than traditional teaching methods. The first two years are primarily basic sciences, and the third and fourth years consist of clinical clerkships and electives. One student says, "The courses here may be just as or more difficult [than undergraduate] but they're also much more interesting and so they don't seem as hard." Students recommend taking histology and liberal arts courses before attending this or any medical school. There is limited competition for grades because it is part of Southern Illinois's philosophy that medical school should not be competitive. Honors are available for any students who deserve them, not just for a predetermined percentage of students.

Immunology, biochemistry, probability, and microbiology are considered to be among the most difficult basic sciences courses. It is stressed that for studying histology, a student should have a diagrammatic representation of what he or she is supposed to be looking for. "Do not take short cuts," adds one student.

The first-year faculty are very available and make a sincere effort to interact with students. The rest of the faculty are slightly more removed from students. There are many research opportunities if you make them for yourself. The school's research policy is currently being revised to make it easier for students to participate in research.

FINANCIAL

The average student spends about $15,000 for a year at Southern Illinois medical school. There are a few scholarships, and most students take out a loan of some sort. It is posssible to work, but not for the average student. The school provides and helps find employment if necessary.

SOCIAL LIFE

There are an average number of social activities for students, including parties, picnics, and intramural sports. Students are relatively low-key and have no reservations about helping each other. As one student says, "The only thing we have in common is a good memory. After that we're all different."

COMMENTS: This school is much more clinically than research oriented. As a result of the changes being made in the teaching techniques, certain courses "do not always flow smoothly. They [Southern Illinois] need to iron out the bumps and creases." One woman adds, "I appreciate the emphasis this school puts on being 'human' doctors. There are some physicians at the school who are great role models. I think the school stands for some of the most fundamental qualities of a good physician, which don't include a high-power research background or a long list of publications. Physicians are human beings helping other human beings."

STANFORD UNIVERSITY
School of Medicine
300 Pasteur Road / Palo Alto, California 94305

LOCATION: Suburban

AGE OF SCHOOL: 80 Years

CONTROL: Private

AMCAS **MEMBER:** Yes

CLASS SIZE: 86

PERCENT WOMEN IN CLASS: 25

PERCENT MINORITIES IN CLASS: 23

AVERAGE STUDENT EXPENDITURE: $$$ (Both in-state and nonresident)

M.D.-Ph.D.: Yes—biochemistry, bioengineering, cancer biology, cell biology, genetics, microbiology, neuroscience, pharmacology, and physiology; also, M.D.-Ph.D. program through Medical Scientist Training Program

NBME **Part I:** Passing grade required for promotion

NBME **Part II:** Passing grade required for graduation

PHYSICAL ENVIRONMENT

Stanford University School of Medicine is located on a main campus that is beautiful by any standards. The Medical Center is surrounded by lush lawns and palm trees. The buildings are modern, and there are many new additions such as the Fairchild Building, a $12 million MRI (Magnetic Resonance Imaging) research facility, and buildings for Molecular Medicine and Genetics. Because of its location on the undergraduate campus, the medical school is a 5- to 10-minute walk or bike ride to undergraduate facilities such as the bookstore, gyms, tennis courts, and a shopping center. Safety does not appear to pose a problem to students here.

It is not difficult to find housing, but the housing surrounding the campus is expensive. Perseverance is strongly recommended because possibilities for cheap housing, such as single rooms in houses, do exist in the area. The school does have dorms for students, but most medical students prefer living off campus. The cost for a one-bedroom apartment is about $400 per month.

Stanford's University Hospital ("very good facilities, up-to-date equipment") is very well maintained, and patients from most SES backgrounds are treated at this facility. Students also rotate out of the Palo Alto VA Hospital, where they are "able to do everything" and have a great deal of hands-on experience. The Kaiser HMO is also considered to be an excellent facility. It is also possible for students to work on an Indian reservation. The variety of health care delivery facilities, ranging from tertiary care hospitals to rural medicine, is astounding. Students feel that they are exposed to "almost every type of patient possible," as well as to a variety of cases ranging from the simplest to those involving the latest technological advances.

ACADEMICS

Stanford students complete their basic sciences the first year and have a flexible clinical curriculum. There are five required disciplines, including pediatrics, psychiatry, obstetrics, medicine, and surgery. Students can take these rotations in any order at any time during the year. It is recommended that prospective students have an adequate science background and take anything and everything besides those science courses required for entrance.

Students are graded on a Pass/Fail option, but as one student phrases it, "Competition lives." Biochemistry is one of the hardest courses encountered by students. The professors are exceptionally warm, and there is a healthy give-and-take between faculty and students. There are more research opportunities available than can be filled. Stanford assists those students who wish to arrange clinical clerkships in foreign countries

FINANCIAL

Stanford will cost the average medical student about $25,000 for the first year. There are numerous job opportunities provided by the school. Students here have mixed emotions about working. Half feel that the money helps them to live better during a stressful time, and the other half feel that working makes the stressful period harder. There are numerous loans and scholarships administered by Stanford medical school.

SOCIAL LIFE

Stanford gives its students the chance to have a good time after they are through working. Students have happy hours, barbecues, and many other social outings during the year. The students at this school have a great sense of humor. They are sharp and witty, and they are certainly not pretentious about their high intellect.

COMMENTS: Stanford University School of Medicine is far more than a "name" school, although its name is synonomous with excellence in medicine. The school has built its outstanding reputation on its innovative curriculum, which allows students to integrate their clinical knowledge with independent research, a caring and nationally recognized faculty, and a gregarious and a heterogeneous student body.

SUNY/BUFFALO
School of Medicine
Farber Hall / Buffalo, New York 14214

LOCATION: Suburban/Medium-Sized City
AGE OF SCHOOL: 142 Years
CONTROL: Public/State

AMCAS **MEMBER:** Yes

SIZE OF CLASS: 138

PERCENT WOMEN IN CLASS: 43

PERCENT MINORITIES IN CLASS: 20

AVERAGE STUDENT EXPENDITURE: $ (In-state); $$ (Nonresident)

M.D.-Ph.D.: Yes—anatomy, biochemistry, biophysics, microbiology, pathology, pharmacology, and physiology

NBME **Part I:** Optional

NBME **Part II:** Optional

PHYSICAL ENVIRONMENT

SUNY/Buffalo School of Medicine is housed in buildings in "very good condition" located in the Health Science Center. The area around the school is suburban ("you can't get a much safer area"). Students say there is no problem with parking and recommend bringing a car to school. The basic sciences and laboratory facilities are very good and spacious.

Buffalo is affiliated with a great number of hospitals, including the recently modernized Buffalo General Hospital ("good equipment and an adequate range of cases and patients"). Children's Hospital offers excellent opportunities for learning pediatric medicine with access to the latest equipment, and it also houses a Rehabilitaion Center. Erie County Medical Center, a major facility for students, houses dialysis centers, a spinal cord injury unit, and inpatient/outpatient services for alcoholism, psychiatric patients, and drug detoxification. Millard Fillmore Hospital houses the Harry M. Dent Neurologic Institute, which has two brain scanners, a computerized pulmonary function laboratory hooked up to five hospitals by telecommunications, a very sophisticated burn unit, and the only civilian hyperbaric chamber in upstate New York. Students find that they are exposed to a wide spectrum of patients through the course of their rotations.

It is not difficult to locate housing at SUNY/Buffalo, and the school provides on-campus accomodations. Students recommend sharing apartments to save money, with the cost of a two-bedroom apartment averaging $150 to $200 per month. Students have easy access to athletic facilities.

ACADEMICS

Buffalo offers its students flexibility with the opportunity to take electives and selectives during the first year. The first two years are devoted primarily to basic and clinical sciences, with electives offered in mathematical, computer, behavioral, and clinical sciences as well as research opportunities. The third year is occupied by participation in clinical clerkships, and the final year is designed by the student.

Competition for grades (Honors/Pass/Fail) is definitely present among students, and one man says, "You can't honestly expect students who were incredibly competitive in college to change overnight. It takes a few semesters for most of the class to 'mellow out.'" It is strongly recommended that prospective students take biochemistry before attending, as well as "anything you just wanted to take but never got around to."

The faculty is not only spoken highly of, but many students say the faculty was one of their major reasons for selecting the school. According to one woman, "They care. I know that sounds trivial. But, when you really need someone to sit down and go over important concepts with you, it really does matter." Buffalo has excellent opportunities for student research.

FINANCIAL

This school is a very good value for New York State residents, who make up most of the class as well as for out-of-staters. The average total cost for the first year is $13,000 for residents and $16,000 for nonresidents. Students take out a combination of various financial aid loans, including ALAS, HEAL, and GSL. There are some jobs for students, and it is felt among students that working is not impossible during the school year.

SOCIAL LIFE

SUNY/Buffalo affords a good variety of social events such as Medical School Follies, Athletic Day, parties, and numerous intramural sports. There are a sizable number of SUNY/Buffalo undergraduates at this school. The students describe their class as outgoing, interesting, and competitive.

COMMENTS: SUNY/Buffalo School of Medicine is an excellent value and has very good clinical facilities, a strong faculty, and a pleasant location (when it is not snowing).

SUNY/STONY BROOK
School of Medicine
Stony Brook, New York 11794

LOCATION: Suburban/Medium-Sized City

AGE OF SCHOOL: 17 Years

CONTROL: Public/State

AMCAS **MEMBER:** No

CLASS SIZE: 100

PERCENT WOMEN IN CLASS: 40

PERCENT MINORITIES IN CLASS: 5

AVERAGE STUDENT EXPENDITURE: $ (In-state); $$ (Nonresident)

M.D.-Ph.D.: Yes—anatomy, biochemistry, microbiology, pathology, pharmacology, and physiology

NBME **Part** I: Students must record a score, which influences promotion.

NBME **Part II:** Students must record a score.

PHYSICAL ENVIRONMENT

The Health Sciences Center (HSC), which houses both SUNY/Stony Brook School of Medicine and the University Hospital, is a futuristic cement-and-glass structure that, in the words of one student, "makes you think you're going to class in a space station on the moon." First-year students attend the majority of their basic sciences classes in the lecture halls in the basement of this immense structure. There are two cafeterias on the first floor and several study rooms built into cement cylinders located near the lecture halls. Lab facilities are maintained in very good condition, and there are "lounging spaces" in the basement floor where students get together before entering the lecture halls.

Students have a wide variety of clinical sites to choose from (often done by lottery system). The University Hospital has excellent facilities and is a top pick for students who do not want to travel very far. Northport VA Hospital offers very good "hands-on" experience and is remarkably well-kept in comparison with other VAs. Long Island Jewish Medical Center gives students more limited exposure to patients.

Stony Brook is a scenic and historic area with many shopping centers, restaurants, and cultural offerings. It is highly recommended that students bring a car, although there is a bus that leaves from the University Hospital and goes to malls and other destinations. There are several area health clubs, and students are able to use athletic facilities on the main campus, which is a three-minute drive away.

Most first-year students chose to live in Chapin (a.k.a. Stage XVI) Apartments and move out into apartments the next year. Chapin is incredibly inexpensive, costing an average of $200 per month, especially when compared to nearby Setauket and Stony Brook itself where one-bedroom apartments easily reach $500 per month. Unfortunately, Chapin is not the most desirable of all living quarters, and for practical purposes, it is difficult to get work done because the walls are paper thin. To combat this, students share houses in the area, which is much less expensive than having an apartment. Students should be advised that they must apply for on-campus housing as soon as possible after receiving their application in the mail.

ACADEMICS

Students believe that the key to success at this medical school is "knowing when to study and when to let steam off." Competition is not that overt because of the Honors/Pass/Fail system, but students are advised not to aim just for minimum passing grades because marginal performance in several courses may result in having to repeat those courses or the entire year. The faculty here are very knowledgeable about their material, and most will go out of their way to accommodate students (particularly in microscopic anatomy). However, there are a few courses students find to be informative but very dry.

There are numerous opportunities for research, and many students take advantage of these, particularly during the summer months when they are off. The curriculum is such that first-year students take basic sciences and spend one day a week at an affiliated hospital under the supervision of a preceptor. Second year continues basic and clinical sciences instruction. The third and fourth years are occupied with clinical clerkships and electives.

When talking about academics, students come back to the same thing over and over; "I feel that they [faculty/administrators] really care if I succeed. It's a really nice feeling especially on days when you have two or more exams."

It is recommended that students take biochemistry because "at times things are glossed over that having had previous exposure might make clearer." Students also feel social sciences and biomedical ethics are good courses to "have under your belt."

FINANCIAL

SUNY/Stony Brook School of Medicine will cost approximately $13,000 for the school year for single, in-state students and $18,000 for nonresidents. The majority of students take out some form of financial aid, including GSLs and NDSL. There are a few job opportunities offered by the school, such as working in the library. Students feel that the first year is too demanding for working outside the classroom.

SOCIAL LIFE

Although SUNY/Stony Brook undergraduate campus is a commuter school and not very active on the weekends, the medical school has its own social life. There are several social functions, including wine and cheese parties held by the school and independent student gatherings such as Big Sib/Little Sib parties. Each entering student is assigned a "Big Sib" who sees that he or she gets old notes, texts, etc. Most students are from New York State, particularly Long Island and the five boroughs.

COMMENTS: It is hard to call Stony Brook an "up and coming" medical school because it has already arrived. Although the school is relatively young, it has accomplished a great deal, including increasing research opportunities and attracting a very strong basic sciences faculty and an outstanding student body. The school offers a quality education in a suburban environment a little more than two hours from New York City.

SUNY/SYRACUSE
(Upstate) Medical Center
College of Medicine
155 Elizabeth Blackwell Street   /   Syracuse, New York 13210

LOCATION: Urban/Medium-Sized City

AGE OF SCHOOL: 154 Years

CONTROL: Public/State

AMCAS **MEMBER:** Yes

CLASS SIZE: 150

PERCENT OF WOMEN IN CLASS: 33

PERCENT OF MINORITIES IN CLASS: 10

AVERAGE STUDENT EXPENDITURE: $ (In-state) $$ (Nonresident)

M.D.-Ph.D.: Yes—available in conjunction with all basic sciences

NBME **Part I:** Students must record a score.

NBME **Part II:** Students must record a score.

PHYSICAL ENVIRONMENT

Upstate Medical Center conducts its basic sciences classes in an older brick building. It has a very modern student center expressly for Health Science Center students. This center has a pool, a basketball court, racquetball courts, extensive weight room facilities, and an area which converts into an auditorium for plays and other activities.

The Syracuse campus has excellent clinical facilities in the State University Hospital ("immaculate and run like a ship"); the VA hospital ("good exposure to patients with multiple medical problems"); Crouse-Irving Memorial Hospital, a major affiliate at which students do much of their OB/GYN rotation; Hutchings Psychiatric Center (most psychiatric training is conducted at this facility); and St. Joseph's Hospital Health Center. The Binghamton campus has the Binghamton General Hospital (excellent intensive care unit here), Our Lady of Lourdes Hospital, and Robert Packer Hospital. Although students consider Syracuse to have a better diversity of patients, Binghamton has the benefit of an innovative approach to clinical clerkships, including the Continuity of Care Program.

The Syracuse complex is located in a safe area, and students do not feel that a car is necessary because the bus system is fairly good. It is recommended that students live in the school's dormitories for at least the first semester because of the large amount of lab work, which is more easily done living on campus. The dorms themselves are in good condition and run about $300 per month. One student felt that living in the dorm made it is easier to meet other students, which is very important particularly if you are new to the area. Apartments in the vicinity of the school average $200 per month plus utilities.

ACADEMICS

SUNY/Syracuse has a sound curriculum that combines both the traditional methodology of medical instruction with a more interdisciplinary approach. The first year is devoted primarily to basic sciences, and students with biochemistry and cell biology are given the chance to take these course in more depth or pursue other interests. Physiology is taught from an organ-systems approach. The primary goal of the school's curriculum is to provide students with a thorough conceptual knowledge of the material rather than forcing them to memorize tremendous amounts of insignificant details. One student cautions, "You still will have a lot of memorizing to do. Particularly in gross anatomy." Students do not have exposure to patients until the second year, when they begin Introduction to Clinical Medicine ("an excellent and informative course").

Grades at SUNY/Syracuse are Honors/Pass/Fail ("very few students get Honors so competition is only intense at the top of the class") with a designated cutoff point (generally a 75 is considered *definitely* passing). The third and fourth year are primarily clinical, and part of the class spends these years in Binghamton. One student comments about this situation; "It can be difficult because you have adjusted to Syracuse and you have to leave for a new place and find new housing." However, students at both Syracuse and Binghamton add that they have excellent clinical training and facilities.

FINANCIAL

The total cost for the first year at SUNY/Syracuse is $13,000 for residents and $16,000 for nonresidents. Most students take out loans of some sort, and the financial aid office is considered to be very helpful. Both students and the administration strongly advise against working due to severe time limitations.

SOCIAL LIFE

The medical school is within easy walking distance of Syracuse University and has its own student activities center. Students have a voice in what goes on at the medical school, and such organizations as the Faculty-Student Association and the Knocker's Society (provides short-term interest-free loans to students) provide input as to the deficiencies in the curriculum. There are also many special interest clubs and intramural sports.

COMMENTS: SUNY/Syracuse is a good medical school with fine clinical facilities. Applicants to this school should be aware of the split campus (Syracuse and Binghamton). Students at this school have very good opportunities for research in areas such as geriatric medicine.

TEMPLE UNIVERSITY
School of Medicine
3400 North Broad Street / Philadelphia, Pennsylvania 19140

LOCATION: Urban/Big City

AGE OF SCHOOL: 87 Years

CONTROL: Private (With state subsidy)

AMCAS MEMBER: Yes

CLASS SIZE: 180

PERCENT WOMEN IN CLASS: 33

PERCENT MINORITIES IN CLASS: 16

AVERAGE STUDENT EXPENDITURE: $$$ (In-state); $$$$ (Nonresident)

M.D.-Ph.D.:   Yes—anatomy, biochemistry, microbiology, pathology, pharmacology, and physiology

NBME Part I: Students must record a score.

NBME Part II: Students must record a score.

PHYSICAL ENVIRONMENT

Temple University School of Medicine is situated in northern Philadelphia and is surrounded by lower SES groups. The basic sciences buildings are fairly new, and the hospital was built within the last three years. The lab/lecture rooms are in good condition and are undergoing some renovation. Library and study facilities are quite good. Students have a separate audiovisual center in the school library that has anatomy dissection videos, biochemistry reviews, and clinical tapes, as well as histology slide carousels that can be viewed on the slide projector in the library.

The hospital sites include Temple University Hospital, a brand-new facility with modern, high-tech equipment (over $11 million worth of new equipment). St. Christopher's Hospital for Children is also a fine facility that houses a unit which helps to assess and treat very young sensorily-damaged children. Albert Einstein Medical Center is a primary clinical site for Temple medical students. There are several other hospital affiliations that include community hospitals, Moss Rehabilitation Center, and the Philadelphia Psychiatric Center. Temple has outstanding clinical facilities, and its students are exposed to a very wide spectrum of patients, cases, and health delivery systems.

The school is near a gym, a basketball court, and racquetball courts , and aerobics classes are available. Very few people live right next to the school, but many students do live about 15 minutes away. Housing is not hard to locate. A two-student apartment (with two bedrooms) averages about $225 per month. One student discusses on-campus housing: "Dorms are available for those desperate, naive, or short-notice admittances, but only as a last choice would I recommend living there."

ACADEMICS

Students strongly recommend taking social sciences such as sociology and psychology before entering medical school. They feel that these courses involve important aspects of the physician/patient relationship. It is also recommended that students take English because writing is a crucial aspect of medicine, especially research writing. Most students here feel that Temple is stronger clinically than in basic sciences.

Almost all students agree that gross anatomy, histology, and embryology (all from the anatomy department) are excellent and well-taught courses. There is a primary care course that runs for four years (primarily first and second years) that discussses ethics, patient-doctor interactions, sexuality, doctors and students as people with problems, and several psychosocial aspects of medicine. There are opportunities for research, but they are not stressed a great deal because of the strong clinical philosophy of the school. However, it should be noted that Temple has extensive research facilities, including the Thrombosis Research Center, The Fels Research Institute for basic studies in carcinogenesis, and through the Skin and Cancer Hospital.

There does not appear to be tremendous competition for grades (Honors/High/Pass/Pass/Condition/Fail) among students, although one student remarks, "It is difficult to rise to the top because everyone is an overachiever." Biochemistry and the third-year medicine rotation are considered the hardest academic disciplines encountered by students. About doing well, one student jokes, "Get extra memory!" Seriously, students point out that organization, after ascertaining the "big picture," is a sound way to study for exams.

FINANCIAL

Temple will cost the average single in-state student about $23,000 and nonresidents about $27,000. Almost everyone at the school uses some form of financial aid. Students feel that lessening costs by leading a spartan existence is not advisable because, as one puts it, "Why make yourself uncomfortable in an already stressful existence?" Students can work between 8 and 10 hours per week, and the school offers a few jobs at lunchtime and after school.

SOCIAL LIFE

There are many things for Temple medical students to do besides study once classes are out. However, most social functions, such as the Friday Night Dance Club, Christmas/talent show, Winter semiformal, and Halloween Costume Party, are not as well attended as could be. Students are not only from varied backgrounds but also from a wide range of ages. Students here are not "cutthroats" but instead are self-motivated, intelligent, and caring. There are several older students at this school who have taken time off after college.

COMMENTS: Temple School of Medicine is an excellent medical school because of its caring faculty and administration and its clinical facilities. Students are very pleased that they chose to attend this school.

TUFTS UNIVERSITY
School of Medicine
136 Harrison Avenue   /   Boston, Massachusetts 02111

LOCATION: Urban/Big City

AGE OF SCHOOL: 136 Years

CONTROL: Private

AMCAS **MEMBER:** Yes

SIZE OF CLASS: 150

PERCENT WOMEN IN CLASS: 30

PERCENT MINORITIES IN CLASS: 3

AVERAGE STUDENT EXPENDITURE: $$$$ (Both in-state and nonresident)

M.D.-Ph.D.: Yes—anatomy and cell biology, biochemistry, immunology, molecular biology and microbiology, neuroscience, and physiology

NBME **Part I:** Passing score required for promotion

NBME **Part II:** Passing score required for graduation

PHYSICAL ENVIRONMENT

Tufts University School of Medicine is located in what is referred to as the Chinatown area of Boston. The school is housed in four modern eight-story buildings. Classroom and laboratory facilities are in "tip-top shape," and students find that the new library (moved in 1986) "more than meets our needs." There are numerous computer-based library searches available, including TOXLINE, MEDLINE, PSYCHINFO, and TAP-IN, a personal information network.

Tufts has excellent clinical facilities. Most students spend a great deal of time at the New England Medical Center Hospitals, which is actually four facilities merged together. The components of the medical center are Boston Dispensary (established in 1796); Boston Floating Hospital for Infants and Children, an outstanding facility that is well run; Pratt Clinic-New England Medical Center; and the Rehabilitation Institute. A new research institute opened up at this facility about two years ago. Baystate Medical Center gives students exposure to middle and upper SES patients and somewhat less autonomy. The Boston VA Medical Center has outstanding opportunities for student research, and St. Elizabeth's Hospital treats both inpatients and outpatients. Students at this school say that they have very good exposure to a wide variety of patients and cases.

The area around Tufts School of Medicine is of questionable safety, and students advise against walking alone after dark. The school is near numerous cultural areas such as Beacon Hill and the theater district. Although the school has dormitory rooms for its students in Posner Hall, students recommend living in apartments away from the school. It is possible to save money by sharing apartments and although housing in Boston is rather expensive students say that shared apartments can be had for between $300 and $400 per month, which is actually considered reasonable by Boston standards.

ACADEMICS

Tufts instituted a new curriculum about three years ago that integrates the study of basic and clinical sciences with other areas, including nutrition, health care economics, and ethics. The program uses problem-based learning, which is based on case studies. The third and fourth years are primarily clinical clerkships with some elective time and opportunities for study abroad. Students recommend a background in biochemistry before attending this school, as well as courses in writing, communications, and psychology.

Competition for grades is moderate, and students recommend being very organized, asking any questions you have while the material is still fresh in your mind, and taking time off whenever you feel overworked, for "You shouldn't study when you know you won't absorb what you're reading." Students find the faculty to be well versed in their subject matter, easily accessible, and interested in what students think about the material covered.

FINANCIAL

Tufts is a costly medical school because of its tuition and because it is located in an expensive city. The total cost for the first year at Tufts is approximately $27,000. Students have a combination of loans, including GSL, ALAS, and HEAL. Working is not recommended by students because of the time constraints involved with the heavy course load. However, there are jobs available in the New England Medical Center that are posted by the financial aid office.

SOCIAL LIFE

This medical school has access to one of the most exciting and historical cities in the United States. Students are involved in many groups, including the Medical Student Council and the Progressive Alliance of Minority Students (PAMS). Students at this school describe their classmates as trustworthy, highly intelligent, and caring.

COMMENTS: Tufts School of Medicine is an outstanding medical school with an innovative curriculum, fine clinical facilities, and a topnotch faculty. Although this is a rather expensive school, students say that it is possible to finance their education through the use of loans and parental and spousal support.

TULANE UNIVERSITY
School of Medicine
1430 Tulane Avenue / New Orleans, Louisiana 70112

LOCATION: Urban/Big City

AGE OF SCHOOL: 154 Years

CONTROL: Private

AMCAS **MEMBER:** Yes

CLASS SIZE: 150

PERCENT WOMEN IN CLASS: 33

PERCENT MINORITIES IN CLASS: 10

AVERAGE STUDENT EXPENDITURE: $$ (In-state); $$$ (Nonresident)

M.D.-Ph.D.: Yes—anatomy, biochemistry, biostatistics, microbiology, parasitology, pharmacology, and physiology

NBME **Part I:** Optional

NBME **Part II:** Optional

PHYSICAL ENVIRONMENT

Tulane Medical Center itself is very new, with state-of-the-art equipment. There are currently plans to increase study facilities for students. There is a weight room on the medical school campus and extensive athletic facilities on the undergraduate campus, which is a 10-minute drive away. The Souchon Museum of Anatomy is an outstanding facility for students. The classrooms are set up nicely, and the library is considered very comfortable for studying.

Tulane has a good number of clinical affiliations, including Tulane Medical Center Hospital ("a very efficient and well-staffed facility"), Charity Hospital, and several other hospitals in New Orleans. Students say that they find they are exposed to a large variety of patients and cases by rotations through the school's clinical sites.

The area surrounding the school is considered relatively safe. Because New Orleans is currently a renter's market, housing is very inexpensive, with a one-bedroom apartment near the school costing from $125 to $175 per month. First-year students often live in dorms to meet other students (particularly if not familiar with the area) and be close to campus, but the dorms are fairly expensive ($350 per month) when compared to off-campus housing. Most students live in apartments and shared houses about 10 to 15 minutes from the school by car.

ACADEMICS

The course work at Tulane School of Medicine is far more demanding than undergraduate science courses due both to volume of material and conceptualization. Students recommend taking biochemistry, histology, and Spanish before entering. Competition for grades (grading system: High Pass/Pass/Conditional/Failure) is not intense. In fact, one student says, "Everyone helps each other. Everyone, the faculty, staff, and students try to make each medical class work as a team." Histology, anatomy, and pharmacology are among the hardest basic sciences encountered by students. It is recommended that students study in groups or pairs with other medical students and try to keep up with the material.

The faculty are praised for both their teaching ability and their accessibility. The school itself is very geared toward students and will do anything possible to help students with problems. Tulane's curriculum allows for electives in the first year as well as Clinical Correlations. The second year continues the study of basic and clinical sciences, and the remaining years are spent doing clinical clerkships and taking electives. There are a great number of research opportunities, which students find easy to obtain and highly rewarding. Students selected Tulane based on its outstanding reputation, its excellent clinical facilities, and the chance to be exposed to a varied group of patients.

FINANCIAL

Tulane will cost about $20,000 for residents and $25,000 for nonresidents for the first year. For students who need to work, Tulane will provide job opporturities for between $6 and $12 per hour working in either the hospital or with a physician. Although these jobs pay reasonably well, students do not recommend working while enrolled, particularly during the first year.

SOCIAL LIFE

"Tulane is in New Orleans. What more social life could you ask for?" Students find ample time for socializing outside the classroom, and there are several organized parties during the course of the year. Students describe their classmates as dependable, down-to-earth, and very friendly.

COMMENTS: This school has the benefits of its location, a curriculum that allows for a degree of freedom and student research, and a strong faculty.

UNIFORMED SERVICES UNIVERSITY OF HEALTH SCIENCE
4301 Jones Bridge Road / Bethesda, Maryland 20814

LOCATION: Big City
AGE OF SCHOOL: 16 Years
CONTROL: Public/Federal
AMCAS **MEMBER:** Yes
CLASS SIZE: 163
PERCENT WOMEN IN CLASS: 20
PERCENT MINORITIES IN CLASS: 10

AVERAGE STUDENT EXPENDITURE: Students are *paid* between $16,000 and $18,000 per year in return for a 7-year committment to armed forces after residency.

M.D.-Ph.D.: No

NBME **Part I:** Students must record a score (test used as a basis for promotion).

NBME **Part II:** Students must record a score (test used as a basis for graduation).

PHYSICAL ENVIRONMENT

Uniformed Services University of Health Sciences (USUHS) is situated on a campus that is about 10 years old. The grounds and facilities are well laid out, with student convenience taken into consideration. The architecture is described as both "comforting" and of "a visually pleasing design." There are many facilities available to students (especially since they are officers) within a short distance (less than a quarter mile) from campus, such as the Naval Officer's Club, the National Naval Medical Center, a swimming pool, three weight rooms, the Armed Forces Radiobiological Research Institute, and the National Institute of Health.

Students rotate out of many well-staffed and relatively modern hospitals, including the Naval Hospital in Bethesda, Walter Reed, and Malcolm Grow Andrews. Students see a variety of patients from several SES groups at these sites. One student comments that the facilities are ultramodern with a great emphasis on minimizing administrative burden on students. There are continual improvements and a high level of maintenance, which ensure very high standards.

Housing in the area of the school is very expensive. One-bedroom apartments in Washington D.C. cost about $550 per month. USUHS students are paid a housing allowance of $250 to $450 per month in addition to military pay. Shared apartments are most common, with shared houses, condos, and townhouses the next preference.

ACADEMICS

The volume of material covered is overwhelming compared to undergraduate school. A high number of "contact hours" (classes are 32 hours per week) creates increased pressure. Recommended courses before attending include comparative anatomy (human if offered), biochemistry, histology, embryology, pathology, and neuroanatomy. All tests are graded objectively, but questions chosen often relate to minutiae. A cooperative spirit exists among students; they are not cutthroat. Gross anatomy is the hardest course encountered by most students at USUHS, with neuroanatomy coming in a close second. Students encourage working in groups in order to share both facts and motivation. Another student suggests making charts and diagrams to help consolidate and solidify the material presented in class.

Many of the faculty at USUHS are from the National Institute of Health, which is just across the street, and they represent the top experts in their respective fields. Student-faculty relationships are good, with faculty available for help outside class. There are numerous opportunities for student research. In fact, several students take a year to conduct research between their second and third years. USUHS has an excellent trauma training program, in which among other things, students are trained to treat battlefield casualties.

FINANCIAL

USUHS is unique in that students are all officers in the Uniformed Services of the United States—with representation in each branch, including Army, Navy, Air Force—or the Public Health Service. Students earn about $18,000 per year in salaried wages and in return are obligated to serve seven years of Active Duty Service. Students are provided with a housing allowance as well as free medical and dental care and commissary privileges. Outside work is not possible at USUHS. Because students are *paid* rather than *pay*, working while attending is not necessary.

SOCIAL LIFE

Students at USUHS are not without a social life. There are bimonthly TGIF parties, a Halloween Party, a School Square Dance, and organized sports and clubs, as well as the vast number of social/cultural offerings available in Washington, D.C. The two major school functions are the Commander's "Dining In" in the fall and the "Dining Out" in the spring. USUHS has little emphasis on military structure. There are no more than one or two inspections per semester. Students here are very outgoing and athletic, and they have a very positive outlook.

COMMENTS: If you are willing to make a military committment after you finish medical school, this is definitely an excellent school to consider. The facilities, location, faculty, and students are all exemplary.

UNIVERSITY OF ARIZONA
College of Medicine
Tuscon, Arizona 85724

LOCATION: Midtown Neighborhood

AGE OF SCHOOL: 21 Years

CONTROL: Public/State

AMCAS **MEMBER:** Yes

CLASS SIZE: 90

PERCENT WOMEN IN CLASS: 33

PERCENT MINORITIES IN CLASS: 10

AVERAGE STUDENT EXPENDITURE: $ (Both in-state and nonresident)

M.D.-Ph.D.: Yes—anatomy, biochemistry, molecular and medical microbiology, pharmacology, and physiology

NBME **Part I:** Students must take and record a score.

NBME **Part II:** Students must take and record a score.

PHYSICAL ENVIRONMENT

The University of Arizona College of Medicine is a modern complex that is part of the Arizona Health Sciences Center. The school was founded in the 1960s, and the buildings are both accessible and close to the main campus (five-minute walk). The school's facilities are modern. However, the rooms where students have their desks, the classrooms, and the library have no windows, which can be distressing to some students.

The school is located in a pleasant midtown neighborhood in Tucson, which is safe for parking cars and bikes. The immediate neighborhood is safe for walking and running. Housing does not appear to be a problem because the medical school's classes start two weeks before those on the main campus. So medical students have a better pick of available housing. The hospital facility is also located so close to the main campus that apartments, small houses, and rooms are fairly easy to find close by.

The major clinical facilities for this school are housed in the University Hospital, which is described as "up to date, well run, [with] a pretty good variety of cases and patients." Another frequently used hospital for rotations is the Tuscon VA Hospital, which is in "good condition and has above-average opportunities for student autonomy." Students feel that they have an adequate variety of patients and cases through the course of their rotations.

Shared apartments are the most common form of housing, and the average cost for a shared apartment is between $200 and $250 dollars per month.

ACADEMICS

The work load is considerably heavier than college, and although the material is not more difficult, the shortened length of time and larger amount of material to master makes it harder than undergraduate. Students felt that the testing and not the material itself was what made it difficult. Arizona's curriculum emphasizes behavioral sciences and provides for patient contact in the first year. The second year consists of more basic and clinical sciences, and the final two years are predominantly clinical clerkships and a large period of time for electives (33 weeks).

Recommendations for courses to take before entering centered on following your own interests. One student felt that prospective students should take Spanish because of the many Hispanic patients they will treat in their future practices.

Tests are graded fairly and competition for grades is not intense because the school uses a Pass/Fail grading system. Many students, however, do not realize that they should try to maintain grades above the mean because the students are ranked.

Anatomy is considered the most difficult course because of the great amounts of memorization in such a short period of time. There are review sessions for anatomy as well as dissecting assignments, which should be kept up with. It is important to obtain copies of old quizzes and exams. They are excellent for reviewing before the actual test. The faculty are very accessible and are eager to help students.

FINANCIAL

For in-state students the cost of attending Arizona medical school will be about $10,000 per year, and for out-of-state students, about $15,000 per year. Almost all students utilize financial aid consisting of loans, scholarships, fellowships, work/study, and grants. It is possible to work during certain semesters, but not recommended during the first semester of the first year or the first year of clinical sciences. Most students work outside the medical college in hospitals and restaurants.

SOCIAL LIFE

There are a great number of social events at Arizona College of Medicine. There are parties such as the Halloween "Cadaver Ball," field trips including camping and river rafting, and football games at which medical students sit together in their own section. In general, the students are friendly, helpful, and supportive of one another.

COMMENTS: This school provides its students with a sound medical program, adequate clinical facilities, and a good faculty.

UNIVERSITY OF CALIFORNIA/DAVIS
School of Medicine
Davis, California 95616

LOCATION: Rural/College Town

AGE OF SCHOOL: 25 Years

CONTROL: Public/State

AMCAS **MEMBER:** Yes

CLASS SIZE: 90

PERCENT WOMEN IN CLASS: 40

PERCENT MINORITIES IN CLASS: 20

AVERAGE STUDENT EXPENDITURE: $ (Both in-state and nonresidents)

M.D.-Ph.D.:   Yes—anatomy, biochemistry, biomedical engine
biophysics, comparative pathology, endocrinology, genetics, mi
nutrition, pharmacology, physiology, and psychology

NBME **Part I:**   Passing score required for promotion

NBME **Part II:**   Students must record a score.

PHYSICAL ENVIRONMENT

University of California Davis medical school buildings are set apart
from the rest of the campus. The buildings are fairly modern and
austere. The surrounding area is flat, and the campus has several
bike paths that serve as major routes of transportation. The school's
facilities are very adequate because the school is relatively new. Students are provided with mailboxes and lockers, as well as microscopes, free of charge.

Davis is a small college town ½ hour from Sacramento, and 1½
hours from San Francisco, and 2 hours from Lake Tahoe and outdoor
areas for skiing and camping. There are several accessible athletic
facilities in the first two years, with a gym and swimming pool within five minutes of the school.

UC/Davis medical school is not next to a hospital and is in a safe
area. There are dormitories for medical students that are considered
"highly liveable." The campus is split up; so students are in Davis
for the first two years and then go to Sacramento, an older medical
complex, for the second two years. Many students move to Sacramento after the second year to avoid the commute. Students should
have a car to get around, but for those who do not, the university
will provide two students with a car to go together to the hospitals.
The Sacramento facility is an urban hospital that houses many Medi-
care patients who cannot travel to other hospitals. The VA Hospital
is very nice, and students like the fact that they do not have weekend
call. Travis Air Force Base is 45 minutes away and is primarily a
military hospital. There is also the Kaiser HMO Hospital, which
treats a wide variety of patients. All the hospitals offer unique opportunities for dealing with a varied group of patients.

It is not difficult to find suitable housing near the school. The
price of a one-bedroom apartment is $300 to $400 per month and a
two-bedroom apartment is $500 to $600 per month. Many apartments are new and have modern conveniences such as dishwashers
and air conditioning. Most students at the school share houses or
apartments.

ACADEMICS

Like the majority of medical and dental students, UC/Davis students do not feel the work itself is much harder than that of undergraduate courses, but there is a far greater amount of material to master. The first year is primarily basic sciences and social sciences, emergency medicine, and a course in relating to patients. Students begin their clinical exposure during the second year, and students do clinical clerkships during the last two years with the opportunity for individualized clinical training during the fourth year.

Biochemistry, microbiology, and humanities courses for stimulation and enjoyment are recommended by students. One student comments, with regard to humanities, "Feed your soul before you have to play this game. There is very little correlation between biochemistry majors and high scores in UCD Medical School biochemistry."

Most exams are multiple-choice. As a result of the letter grade system employed by the school, students are competitive for higher grades. Microbiology, gross anatomy, and pharmacology are considered among the more difficult courses encountered during the first two years of basic sciences. Students recommend not cramming and occasionally cutting lectures to allow yourself to learn the material. The faculty are considered very caring and excellent educators. There are good opportunities for student research at this school.

FINANCIAL

UC/Davis has the advantage of being a state school with both low tuition and reasonable living expenses. The cost for a year for an in-state single student will be about $10,000; $15,000 for nonresidents. Loans and tight budgets are a must for most students. Students do not feel it is practical to work at this school unless there is no other way of attending.

SOCIAL LIFE

Diverse best sums up the students found at this medical school. The school has Ph.D. physiologists and construction workers together in the same class. Many students here are older, and there is a high percentage of women in the class. Students schedule parties for themselves, and there are wine and cheese parties given by the school. One professor in particular is always willing to host large parties at his ranch. The work load at this school is heavy, to say the least, but students form their own support groups and help each other to become competent, caring physicians.

COMMENTS: UC/Davis has an excellent minority recruitment program and is favorable to older applicants who have taken time off before entering medical school. This school takes painstaking efforts to make sure its students are accommodated both in and outside the classroom. It has very good clinical facilities, a caring faculty and administration, and is an excellent value, particularly for California residents.

UNIVERSITY OF CALIFORNIA/LOS ANGELES
School of Medicine
Los Angeles, California 90024

LOCATION: Urban/Big City

AGE OF SCHOOL: 42 Years

CONTROL: Public/State

AMCAS **MEMBER:** Yes

SIZE OF CLASS: 165

PERCENT WOMEN IN CLASS: 50

PERCENT MINORITIES IN CLASS: N/A

AVERAGE STUDENT EXPENDITURE: $ (In-state); $$ (Nonresident)

M.D.-Ph.D.: Yes—anatomy, biological chemistry, biology, biomathematics, experimental pathology, immunology, medical physics and radiology, microbiology, molecular biology, neurosciences, pharmacology, and physiology; also available through Medical Scientist Training Program; also, combined M.D.-Master of Public Health (M.P.H.) available, as well as combined 7-year biomedical program with UC/Riverside and Harbor-UCLA Medical Center

NBME **Part I:** Students must take as a candidate, and scores are considered for promotion and graduation.

NBME **Part II:** Students must take as a candidate, and scores are considered for promotion and graduation.

PHYSICAL ENVIRONMENT

The University of California/Los Angeles (UCLA) medical center is very big: "The first thing that strikes you about it is the size. This place is so large it's overwhelming." The medical school is located in the Center for Health Sciences, and students find the basic sciences instructional and laboratory facilities to be in very good condition. The area around the school is considered safe. The campus is quite attractive, and the school itself is close to Westwood, which is a nice area, with its restaurants and shopping, for taking a breather after classes.

UCLA has very strong clinical facilities, including the University Hospital ("very well staffed, modern equipment") and Harbor General, the Brain Research Institute, the Jerry Lewis Neuromuscular Research Center, the Jules Stein Eye Institute, and the Neuropsychiatric Institute and Hospital ("an oustanding hospital with great rehabilitation facilities"). UCLA also has one of the eight hospital-based biomedical cyclotrons in the United States. There are numerous other affiliations that provide students with an enormous variety of patients and cases.

It can be difficult to find reasonably priced housing near the medical school because the surrounding areas are expensive. Students say the average cost of a one-bedroom apartment is between $550 and $750 per month. Sharing rooms is seen as the logical solution to the exorbitant housing costs. There is a 12-month waiting list for on-campus housing.

ACADEMICS

Students begin their exposure to patients in the first year by learning H&Ps (Histories & Physicals). The advanced basic sciences courses are taught by an organ-system approach during the second year. Students rotate through clinical clerkships the third year and take electives their final year at UCLA. "Competition is definitely intense the first year." (Letter grades are used for basic sciences.) Students strongly recommend taking biochemistry, economics, and any courses that will "make you a more well-rounded physician."

The faculty are highly regarded, although some students find them somewhat distant. There are outstanding opportunities for student research through formal M.D.-Ph.D. programs and individual accommodations. Students have no "set method" for academic success other than "sticking with it and do not give up!"

FINANCIAL

UCLA is a very reasonably priced medical school for
dents, with the total cost of the first year coming to $
dents and $16,000 for nonresidents. Students take ou
that working is not possible while enrolled at this school.

SOCIAL LIFE

"If you're going to study as long we have to, you got to let yourself
go once in a while." Students at this school have relatively active
social lives outside the classroom. There are student functions and
students say that "hanging out with fellow students" is a favorite
pastime.

COMMENTS: UCLA combines a thorough basic and clinical sciences preparation with outstanding clinical facilities. This is an excellent medical school for applicants to consider.

UNIVERSITY OF CALIFORNIA/SAN DIEGO
School of Medicine
La Jolla, California 92093

LOCATION: Suburban/Medium-Sized City

AGE OF SCHOOL: 20 Years

CONTROL: Public/State

AMCAS **MEMBER:** Yes

SIZE OF CLASS: 120

PERCENT WOMEN IN CLASS: 35

PERCENT MINORITIES IN CLASS: 25

AVERAGE STUDENT EXPENDITURE: $ (Both in-state and nonresident)

M.D.-Ph.D.: Yes—bioengineering, biology, chemistry, neurosciences,
pathology, physiology, and pharmacology

NBME **Part I:** Passing score required for promotion

NBME **Part II:** Students must record a score.

PHYSICAL ENVIRONMENT

The University of California/San Diego (USD) medical school is made up of relatively new buildings that are clean, modern, and well maintained. The medical school is located on the main campus and is a 5- to 10-minute walk to campus facilities such as athletic equipment. The clinical facilities are excellent and there is an entire building for oncology and another for MRI (Magnetic Resonance Imaging). The hospital sites are extremely varied, ranging from a health maintenance organization (Kaiser) to rural care facilities in northern California and the chance to work on an Indian reservation or in a major tertiary care medical center (UCSD Medical Center). Students find that they are exposed to a variety of patients, cases, and types of health care delivery facilities.

The school is situated in La Jolla on a cliff that overlooks miles of beaches. Housing is not difficult to locate due in part to the good housing office and many listings. But start looking well in advance of when classes are scheduled to begin. Costs are moderate, with housing near the campus costing between $350 and $400 per month. There is a one-year waiting list for on-campus housing.

ACADEMICS

UCSD's curriculum is highly innovative and allows students to meet their individual learning needs. The first year consists of basic and clinical sciences with elective time, biostatistics, and behavioral sciences. Anatomy is taken during the second year along with electives, and the last two years are occupied with clinical clerkships and electives. Students do not find that there is much competition for grades (Pass/Fail and narrative reports).

Students recommend taking biochemistry, some physiology, and cell biology and having a familiarity with computers before entering. It is stressed that to be most successful students should understand the concepts rather than cram and/or try to memorize every detail.

FINANCIAL

UCSD is an excellent value for Californians (tuition is only $400 per quarter). The total cost for residents is about $10,000, with nonresidents spending $15,000 per year. There are some minor jobs available, but students feel that it is not easy to work while enrolled at this school.

SOCIAL LIFE

According to one student, there are about three or four "official parties" per quarter and one "unofficial party" per week. Students at
this school have numerous social events, including TGIF parties, talent shows, ski trips, golf tournaments, and intramural sports. The
class is very diversified. One students describes his classmates as
"very Californian . . . fun and smart."

COMMENTS: One student adds these additional points about
UCSD: "Many people are concerned about the requirement for independent study projects at UCSD. They should be aware that the
required research can be in any aspect of medicine including cultural,
historical, clinical, theoretical, etc. We have good opportunities for
contact with patients early on. The exposure is mostly observational
but is still rewarding." Another student says, "La Jolla [San Diego]
is the premiere place for a medical school. The area is beautiful,
sunny 90 percent of the time, no inner city or anything. The faculty
and staff are very helpful and there is a desire to make sure everyone
gets through. Just plain too much fun!"

UNIVERSITY OF CALIFORNIA/SAN FRANCISCO
School of Medicine
San Francisco, California 94143

LOCATION: Big City

AGE OF SCHOOL: 124 Years

CONTROL: Public/State

AMCAS **MEMBER:** Yes

CLASS SIZE: 141

PERCENT WOMEN IN CLASS: 42

PERCENT MINORITIES IN CLASS: 45

AVERAGE STUDENT EXPENDITURE: $ (Both in-state and nonresident)

M.D.-Ph.D.:   Yes—anatomy, biochemistry, bioengineering, health psychology, immunology, medical anthropology, microbiology, pathology, pharmacology, and physiology; also, M.D.-Masters of Public Health (MPH) and M.D.-M.S. joint program between UC/Berkeley and UC/San Francisco

NBME **Part I:**   Passing grade required for promotion

NBME **Part II:**   Students must record a score.

PHYSICAL ENVIRONMENT

University of California/San Francisco School of Medicine is housed on the health sciences campus, which several students describe as "a very exciting environment to be learning medicine in because of the large number of students enrolled in the health professions assembled in one campus." The basic sciences are taught in the Medical Sciences Building, which is considered more than adequate in terms of classrooms and laboratories. Athletic facilities, including the Milberry Gymnasium, which has a pool, weights, racquetball, and Ping-Pong, are readily available.

There have been some problems with safety in the area of the school in past years, although this issue is being addressed by students and the administration. It can be somewhat difficult to locate suitable housing near the school. An average one-bedroom apartment near the school costs about $450 per month. Apartments are the most common form of housing. Students feel that having a car would definitely be beneficial, but it is not absolutely necessary because public transportation is available.

Certainly, one of the strongest features of this medical school is its extensive clinical facilities. Between rotations in the VA Hospital, the University Hospital, Mount Zion Hospital, and affiliations with 33 other hospitals, students here find that they have exposure to an incredible spectrum of patients from every SES and excellent opportunities to work in a variety of health care delivery facilities that see cases ranging from the simplest to those requiring the most sophisticated procedures in medicine.

ACADEMICS

This school also has the advantage of a highly innovative and flexible curriculum that allows the student to choose in what order he or she will take the required courses and has an outstanding number and variety of elective courses. The first year consists primarily of basic sciences. Students strongly recommend taking biochemistry and immunology prior to attending this school. Students have their first experience with patients during the first year in Introduction to Clinical Medicine (ICM). The second year continues the study of basic sciences along with clinical and social sciences. Third year is primarily clinical clerkships, and the fourth year consists of choosing from among seven "Pathways," which include medical scientist, surgical, general, behavioral specialist, social and administrative, and research.

The faculty at this school are highly praised by students as "leaders in medical education in both the clinic and in research. But, the best part is that they really care about students and take the time out of their busy schedules to meet with you if you have a question." Competition for good grades (grading system: Pass/Not Pass) is all but nonexistent, and students feel that cooperation is the key to success. This school actively encourages research, and students have numerous opportunities ranging from research in clinical and basic sciences to research in foreign countries.

FINANCIAL

This school is an outstanding value for both Californians and nonresidents alike. The total cost for the first year is $11,000 for residents and $15,000 for nonresidents. San Francisco has an excellent financial aid office, and most students take out a combination of loans over the four years. Students strongly advise against working because of the time constraints that medical school places on them.

SOCIAL LIFE

Students at this school say that having a social life is a very individual decision at this school. For those interested in socializing, there are numerous cultural and entertainment facilities in the vicinity of the school. The word *diverse* cannot begin to describe the incredible variety of students attending this medical school, including a considerable number of nonresidents.

COMMENTS: There are several reasons this school has gained a reputation as one of the leading medical schools in the country. UC/San Francisco has outstanding clinical facilities and affiliations (this is not debatable), the faculty are nationally recognized for their research and advances in medicine (along with this they are also very good teachers and conveyers of information), and the curriculum is flexible, allowing students numerous opportunities for research if they so choose. Another important aspect of this school is that it has an exemplary record for minority applicant recruitment.

UNIVERSITY OF CINCINNATI
College of Medicine
231 Bethesda Avenue / Cincinnati, Ohio 45267

LOCATION: Urban/Big City

AGE OF SCHOOL: 169 Years

CONTROL: Public/State

AMCAS **MEMBER:** Yes

CLASS SIZE: 150

PERCENT WOMEN IN CLASS: 33

PERCENT MINORITIES IN CLASS: 5

AVERAGE STUDENT EXPENDITURE: $$ (Both in-state and nonresident)

M.D.-Ph.D.: Yes—anatomy, biochemistry, cell biology, developmental biology, environmental health, microbiology, molecular biology, molecular genetics, pathology and laboratory medicine, pharmacology and cell biophysics, and physiology

NBME **Part I:** Passing score required for promotion to the fourth year

NBME **Part II:** Students must record a score.

PHYSICAL ENVIRONMENT

The University of Cincinnati College of Medicine is located in the Medical Sciences building, which is a national center for medical research. The school is housed in a new nine-story building attached to the teaching hospital and is affiliated with six hospitals within walking distance, including one of the best children's hospitals in the area. The building has a small weight room and is about a mile from the main campus. The facilities are constantly being updated as a result of the fact that the staff in the medical research building are on the "cutting edge" of medical research. This building was the largest building devoted to medical research in the United States at the time it was built.

The school is in an urban area surrounded primarily by lower SES family housing. Inexpensive housing is easy to locate if you look at the "right time." Students suggest looking for apartments and shared houses, which are the major source of student housing, between May and June. Prices for apartments vary greatly, ranging from $120 to $400 per month. The area surrounding the school is reasonably safe if proper cautions are taken at night, such as walking in groups.

ACADEMICS

One student compares the work here to college in the following way: "In [undergraduate courses] you studied for the test. Here you have to *learn* and remember." It is recommended that prospective students take histology, biochemistry, and comparative anatomy before attending this school. Competition for good grades is intense, but aside from a small group at the top of the class, there is a lot of "information sharing." Histology and gross anatomy are among the hardest basic sciences for students.

Outlining the chapters in the texts helps students to retain the information and makes it easier to refer to. A student adds, "The key here is to know all the facts and see how they relate to one another." The faculty at this school go out of their way to help students, particularly the biochemistry department, which meets with students over lunch to get feedback on the progress of the courses. There are several opportunities for research, primarily over the summer. Some of the main reasons students chose this school were its reputation, its cost, and the fact that there is early exposure to patients.

FINANCIAL

Cincinnati will cost a total of approximately $17,000 for in-state residents and $20,000 for nonresidents. Students find that loans here are essential, and many students have taken military scholarships. There are some smaller jobs available for students, but working is not recommended during the first year.

SOCIAL LIFE

This school tries to make the transition from college to medical school a smooth one. For this reason, a group of first-year students (usually six) and the same number of second-year medical students are put into a "support group." This group forms a support/social network for each student. Some groups have Sunday brunches together, play intramural sports, and have potluck dinners. Most social activities are planned by students, such as the Pub Crawl (buses full of medical students going from bar to bar), ski trips, and a Bahamas party. Students selected the school because, as one student says, "The faculty and students are people—not machines/eggheads/gunners." Most students agree that one of the best things about their school is the well-roundedness of the students it attracts.

COMMENTS: One student says about the University of Cincinnati College of Medicine, "The school runs like a well-oiled machine. Departments (i.e. biochemistry and anatomy) work together so a student doesn't have two tests within hours/days of each other. . . . Free tutoring is available to anyone who needs it. The Student Affairs Office treats students like they own the place. The general secretary (known as Iva Dean) is a wizard with paperwork/financial aid red tape. . . . You can really feel comfortable here."

UNIVERSITY OF CONNECTICUT
School of Medicine
Farmington Avenue / Farmington, Connecticut 06032

LOCATION: Suburban/Small City

AGE OF SCHOOL: 25 Years

CONTROL: Public/State

AMCAS **MEMBER:** Yes

SIZE OF CLASS: 88

PERCENT WOMEN IN CLASS: 50

PERCENT MINORITIES IN CLASS: 10

AVERAGE STUDENT EXPENDITURE: $ (In-state); $$ (Nonresident)

M.D.-Ph.D.: Yes—cell biology, developmental biology, immunology, molecular biology, neuroscience, pharmacology, physiology, and toxicology

NBME **Part I:** Students must record a score, which is used to determine final course grades.

NBME **Part II:** Students must record a score.

PHYSICAL ENVIRONMENT

The University of Connecticut (UCONN) School of Medicine is housed in a beautiful and modern structure in a suburban area that is "breathtakingly beautiful in the fall with the foliage." The basic sciences and laboratory facilities (MDLs—multidisciplinary laboratories) are modern and are considered very good. UCONN is surrounded by a rather safe area; few students have had any problems with safety. It is recommended that students bring a car to campus.

UCONN has adequate hospital facilities including the University Hospital ("very modern, up-to-date equipment, and outstanding nursing staff") and 10 other affiliated hospitals. Students feel that they receive a fair variety of patients and cases through the course of their rotations.

Getting reasonably priced housing near the school can be difficult, but one student says you can find somewhat inexpensive housing if you look early enough. The average cost for a shared apartment is $250 per month, although there is a great deal of more expensive housing that is close to the campus. There are no athletic facilities at this school, which is 40 minutes away from the Storrs (main) Campus. But students say there is a discount at the local Jewish Community Center.

ACADEMICS

It is strongly recommended that students take biochemistry, psychology, and writing courses before attending this medical school. Students find the academic environment to be "cooperative due to the Pass/Fail grading system." However, there is some competition because passing is determined by how well the class scores.

The faculty range from very poor teachers and excellent researchers to very excellent researchers and conveyers of information. Overall, the faculty are very receptive and approachable, particularly the deans, who "almost side with student opinion for proposed changes." There are several research opportunities for students, although it is pointed out that these opportunities pay very poorly.

UCONN's curriculum is innovative in that students are exposed to clinical medicine from the first month and courses are taught using an interdisciplinary approach. More advanced basic sciences are taught by using an organ-systems approach the second year, and the third and fourth years are occupied by clinical clerkships and electives. It is imporant to study independently with the supplied syllabus, obtain old tests when possible, and learn what lectures not to attend.

FINANCIAL

The average cost of UCONN is about $13,000 for residents and $18,000 for nonresidents. Most students take out GSLs and the school's low interest loans, but few resort to HEALs. The school offers low-paying work opportunities, so students are advised to seek employment in the community in order to make more money.

SOCIAL LIFE

Although isolated from the undergraduate campus, UCONN medical students have many opportunities for a social life. The school has advocacy groups, "Ad Groups," for first- and second-year students to help them adjust to medical school. There are numerous organizations, such as the Health Center Players, which puts on theatrical productions, the Film Society, and AMSA. The Gong Show is a talent show put on by UCONN students, and each January there is a Dressed to Kill party. Students describe their class as a "mixed bunch, dedicated, caring, and supportive of each other."

COMMENTS: UCONN is a good value for Connecticut residents. The school's basic sciences instructional and lab facilities are very good, and the curriculum is highly innovative. Overall, this is a good medical program.

UNIVERSITY OF FLORIDA
College of Medicine
J. Hillis Miller Health Center / Gainesville, Florida 32610

LOCATION: Medium-Sized City

AGE OF SCHOOL: 32 Years

CONTROL: Public/State

AMCAS **MEMBER:** Yes

SIZE OF CLASS: 114

PERCENT WOMEN IN CLASS: 44

PERCENT MINORITIES IN CLASS: 7

AVERAGE STUDENT EXPENDITURE: $ (Both in-state and nonresident)

M.D.-Ph.D.: Yes—anatomy, biochemistry, immunology, medical microbiology, neuroscience, pathology, pharmacology, and physiology

NBME **Part I:** Passing score required for graduation

NBME **Part II:** Passing score required for graduation

PHYSICAL ENVIRONMENT

The overall appearance of the J. Hillis Miller Health Center and Shands Teaching Hospital is that of a large and modern hospital. There are older sections, including underground walkways between the buildings, but the student labs, classrooms, and much of the hospitals are new or have been recently renovated. Students find that they are exposed to an adequate variety of patients and cases through the clinical facilities, including Shands Teaching Hospital and the nearby VA Hospital.

The health center is approximately three blocks from the heart of the University of Florida campus. The campus houses several athletic facilities, including indoor and outdoor pools, tracks, tennis courts, and modern gyms. Gainesville is a good sized city of about 120,000 people. The hospital area is surrounded by the University of Florida campus to the south and a mixture of farms and apartment complexes on the other sides.

It is not difficult to find housing in the vicinity of the hospital. One bedroom apartments range from $200 to $300 per month. Two-bedroom apartments cost between $300 and $400 per month depending on location and facilities. Renting larger houses is considered to be one of the best types of student housing because it is usually cheaper than renting apartments when the cost of the house is shared by a group of students.

ACADEMICS

"Take biochemistry!" Students strongly recommend having a solid foundation in the basic and social sciences, including courses in biochemistry, histology, psychology, and sociology. Competition for grades is moderate, and one woman adds, "We compete against each other, but we're always willing to help another student who needs it." The faculty are considered very good communicators, and are sympathetic to student problems.

The curriculum is primarily traditional, with courses in human behavior and medical ethics the first year (in addition to basic sciences). U. Florida has adequate research opportunities for students. It is stressed that keeping up with course work is the key to academic success. "Do a little (actually at this school it's a lot) at a time and you'll do just fine."

FINANCIAL

The cost for the first year is about $10,000 for residents and $15,000 for nonresidents. Students take out a variety of loans and feel that working is possible after the first year.

SOCIAL LIFE

Florida has a good social life, and students are involved in several organizations. Students have diverse backgrounds and a wide variety of interests. They describe their class as "caring, smart but not pompous, and self-sufficient."

COMMENTS: U. Florida has the benefits of a good location and good preclinical facilities. The faculty are very good, and the student body is highly motivated.

UNIVERSITY OF HAWAII
John A. Burns School of Medicine
1960 East-West Road / Honolulu, Hawaii 96822

LOCATION: Big City

AGE OF SCHOOL: 23 Years

CONTROL: Public/State

AMCAS **MEMBER:** Yes

CLASS SIZE: 57

PERCENT WOMEN IN CLASS: 35

PERCENT MINORITIES IN CLASS: N/A

AVERAGE STUDENT EXPENDITURE: $ (In-state); $$$ (Nonresident)

M.D.-Ph.D.: Yes—biochemistry, genetics, pharmacology, physiology, reproductive biology, and tropical medicine

NBME **Part I:** Passing score required for promotion

NBME **Part II:** Passing score required for graduation

PHYSICAL ENVIRONMENT

The John A. Burns School of Medicine is located in a relatively new building stylized to resemble an Oriental pagoda and surrounded by trees and grass. All campus facilities are within walking distance of the medical school. The medical school is relatively safe, although women should probably not walk alone at night. Medical students have free access to athletic facilities as long as they have a valid ID The medical school facilities are adequate, and each student is provided with his or her own study carrel for the first two years. These carrels are open 24 hours a day, 7 days a week, which makes them very convenient for students.

Hawaii medical school students rotate out of many hospitals, including Kapliania Red and Queens hospitals, which are both in good condition. St. Francis is an older hospital in adequate condition that has many older patients in for dialysis. Tripler Army Hospital is a fine facility that has many military patients and their families. There is a definite clinical emphasis at this school, which students enjoy greatly.

The University of Hawaii is located at the base of Manoa Valley, and the school gets a great deal of rain. Manoa is part of the city of

Honolulu. Housing is fairly hard to find and also quite expensive. A one-bedroom apartment costs between $500 and $575 per month. Sharing an apartment is the best choice. Those in search of less expensive housing may use student dormitories, but they have to contend with the noisy undergraduates who share the dormitories.

ACADEMICS

Courses at Hawaii medical school are more difficult than undergraduate courses, but the information is more interesting, which makes the courses easier to study for. Students recommend technical writing and speed reading to prospective students. Competition is kept to a minimum because grading is Pass/Fail. Pathology and gross anatomy are among the hardest courses here.

Studying in small groups and keeping up so that you have a second chance to see the material will help students succeed at this school. There are numerous opportunities for research. The faculty are considered very good, and most are accessible to students.

FINANCIAL

The University of Hawaii medical school will cost a single in-state student living in an apartment a little over $13,000 for the school year (as opposed to $23,000 for nonresidents). Loans are a must for most students, and the financial aid office is very helpful to students in need of assistance. It is possible to work while attending here, but it is not recommended during the first year.

SOCIAL LIFE

There are many social activities sponsored by the University of Hawaii, more so from the undergraduate campus than the medical school. There is an annual luau for the seniors given by the first-year class, as well as concerts and plays. The class is friendly, close, and supportive.

COMMENTS: Students at this school find that they are able to relax from the rigors of their courses in the peaceful setting outside school. Hawaii is reasonably priced for residents and has a very good faculty.

UNIVERSITY OF IOWA
College of Medicine
100 College of Medicine Administration Building   /   Iowa City, Iowa 52242

LOCATION: Medium-Size City

AGE OF SCHOOL: 138 Years

CONTROL: Public/State

AMCAS **MEMBER:** Yes

CLASS SIZE: 175

PERCENT WOMEN IN CLASS: 30

PERCENT MINORITIES IN CLASS: 15

AVERAGE STUDENT EXPENDITURE: $ (In-state); $$ (Nonresident)

M.D.-Ph.D.: Yes—anatomy, biochemistry, community medicine, microbiology, pharmacology, and physiology

NBME **Part I:** Optional

NBME **Part II:** Optional

PHYSICAL ENVIRONMENT

University of Iowa College of Medicine is made up of new modern additions tastefully added to the gothic architecture of the hospital. Clustered around the teaching hospital are well-equipped modern basic sciences buildings. There is a large student recreation center that has a pool, basketball and racquetball courts, and other facilities, adjacent to the University Hospital. Downtown, complete with stores and theaters, is a five-minute walk from the school. The area surrounding the school is perceived as moderately safe.

The school's basic sciences facilities are very modern, with a new five-story research facility under construction. The hospital is primarily modern with a few remaining older areas still being used. The labs are readily available on a comprehensive hospital computer system. Iowa medical school is located in an area which exposes its students to a large rural patient population.

Housing is currently a renter's market, with a wide variety of houses and apartments near the hospital. Housing is reasonable, with a two-bedroom apartment costing about $350 to $400 per month.   Family housing for married couples or single parents is available for less than $200 per month.

ACADEMICS

Conceptually the material is not much harder than undergraduate courses, but the volume is much heavier. Students feel that prospective students should pursue their own interests whether they be sciences or humanities. There is no ranking system for students, and the grading system is Honors/Pass/Fail so that most students tend to compete against themselves rather than each other.

Biochemistry and microbiology are considered very difficult because of the sheer volume of information that the courses entail. Organization and discipline are crucial to succeeding, as well as keeping up on a day-to-day basis. The basic faculty are considered somewhat distant by students. However, the clinical instructors are more open with students and are very concerned with student needs. There are many research opportunities, and research is encouraged by the school. Many students pursue summer research opportunities or combined M.D.-Ph.D. degrees.

FINANCIAL

In-state, single students pay about $14,000 for the total year, while nonresidents pay about $20,000. Loans are considered a must to most students here, with GSLs, HPSLs, and HEALs playing a large part in financing. Some students hold part-time jobs, but very few. A number of positions are available at the hospital including EKG technicians and blood gas and phlebotomy teams. These openings are usually filled by word of mouth.

SOCIAL LIFE

Students at Iowa medical school are highly motivated and also place a high value on extracurricular activities. There are many social events planned for students, including waltzes, formal banquets, and informal parties. Students are concerned with their school's future.

COMMENTS: Iowa College of Medicine has strong research and clinical facilities as well as a very dynamic faculty.

UNIVERSITY OF LOUISVILLE
School of Medicine
Health Sciences Center / Louisville, Kentucky 40292

LOCATION: Urban/Medium-Sized City

AGE OF SCHOOL: 155

CONTROL: Public/State

AMCAS **MEMBER:** Yes

CLASS SIZE: 124

PERCENT WOMEN IN CLASS: 30

PERCENT MINORITIES IN CLASS: 2

AVERAGE STUDENT EXPENDITURE: $ (In-state); $$$ (Nonresident)

M.D.-Ph.D.: Yes—anatomy, biochemistry, biophysics, immunology, microbiology, pharmacology, physiology, and toxicology

NBME **Part I:** Passing score required for promotion

NBME **Part II:** Optional

PHYSICAL ENVIRONMENT

University of Louisville medical school is a complex of modern concrete buildings. The school is in a downtown location and is surrounded by a relatively high crime area. The main campus (Belknap) is several miles from the medical school and has athletic equipment including a gym, swimming pool, and track. There is a weight room in the basement of the medical school. Although there is a bus system downtown, it is recommended that students have a car.

The school buildings are fairly new (built in the 1970s), and the main teaching hospital was built in 1983. The facilities are relatively modern, but they lack computers. There is planned renovation, including the expanding of office space. There are three main hospital facilities out of which students rotate. The VA Hospital is a little run down and houses a normal mixture of elderly veteran patients. The University Hospital is now a Humana hospital and caters to private patients. It has the best facilities of any hospital site at the school. Trober Clinic provides students with a stipend and housing.

Finding suitable housing is no problem at Louisville medical school. Housing can be obtained within a five-minute car ride and is relatively inexpensive. The average cost for a one-bedroom apartment is between $200 and $300 per month. Most students live in apartments.

ACADEMICS

"Eat, drink, and sleep these courses and if provided with a good text book, read it!" This is the advice of one Louisville student on how to succeed at this school. The level of difficulty of courses is the same as undergraduate, but the amount of information is greatly increased. Students strongly recommend taking a "good histology course if offered and biochemistry courses." Everyone here tries for their individual best but in a way that does not foster overt competition.

Gross anatomy is considered to be among the hardest basic sciences courses. There is open communication between students and faculty. The faculty are always available for help and will schedule reviews if requested. Summer fellowship and research opportunities in general are abundant. Students find that the school is much stronger in clinical instruction than in basic sciences. The school has an excellent reputation in surgical instruction.

FINANCIAL

Louisville costs about $15,000 for in-state students and $22,000 for out-of-staters. The dean's office is reputed to be very helpful in assisting students with locating financial aid. The school does not allow freshmen to work, but it is possible for upperclassmen to work about four or five hours per week. Most students take out GSLs, with a good number also utilizing HEALs.

SOCIAL LIFE

Students have a formal that is known as the "Cadaver Ball." There are also many social events, including a class picnic, golf and football tournaments, and post-test parties. Students describe their classmates as "very friendly, helping people. A very diverse group."

COMMENTS: Louisville has expanded its clinical facilities and has good opportunities for student research. However, the school is somewhat more clinically than research oriented.

UNIVERSITY OF MARYLAND
School of Medicine
655 West Baltimore Street / Baltimore, Maryland 21201

LOCATION: Urban/Big City

AGE OF SCHOOL: 180 Years

CONTROL: Public/State

AMCAS **MEMBER:** Yes

CLASS SIZE: 152

PERCENT WOMEN IN CLASS: 33

PERCENT MINORITIES IN CLASS: 7

AVERAGE STUDENT EXPENDITURE: $ (In-state); $$ (Nonresident)

M.D.-Ph.D.: No

NBME **Part I:** Students must take exam (scores influence promotion and certain course grades).

NBME **Part II:** Students must take exam (score influence graduation).

PHYSICAL ENVIRONMENT

The University of Maryland School of Medicine is made up of a mixture of buildings, most of which are fairly new. There is no campus per se. The medical school is very close to the student gym, and the hospital is attached to the class building. It is a very compact inner city campus.

Maryland has very good clinical facilities, including the University Hospital ("a very academic atmosphere and also well run") and several hospitals in Baltimore. Multiple renovations, such as a new trauma center, are being made in the hospital. There is also the Sudden Infant Death Syndrome Institute.

Surrounding the school is a tough inner city neighborhood. Housing around the school is easily found. There are several renovated townhouses in the area. Rent is not very high, with average rents being about $200 per month for an apartment. Many medical students choose to share houses.

ACADEMICS

Students begin their introduction to the clinic in the first year with Introdution to Clinical Practices. The second year is primarily advanced basic sciences using an organ-systems approach, while the remaining two years are occupied by clinical clerkships and electives. Students recommend taking humanities and the basic premedical requirements before attending because you will "never have such a good opportunity to learn about these areas." Competition is not that overwhelming, and students find pathology and gross anatomy to be among the most challenging basic sciences.

The clinical faculty are considered stronger than their basic sciences counterparts. There are numerous opportunities for student research. Students recommend "staying on top of the work" for academic success.

FINANCIAL

The average cost for the first year at this school is $14,000 for residents and $20,000 for nonresidents. Students say the financial aid office is very good. Most take out some form of loan. Working is nearly impossible, particularly during the first year.

SOCIAL LIFE

There are a few opportunities for social interaction, and the class has faculty-student happy hours. The student body at this school is diverse, and members are close to one another.

COMMENTS: Maryland medical school has good clinical facilities, an excellent clinical faculty, and several opportunities for student research.

UNIVERSITY OF MASSACHUSETTS
Medical School
55 Lake Avenue, North / Worcester, Massachusetts 01605

LOCATION: Medium-Sized City
AGE OF SCHOOL: 26 Years

CONTROL: Public/State

AMCAS **MEMBER:**   Yes

CLASS SIZE: 100

PERCENT WOMEN IN CLASS: 42

PERCENT MINORITIES IN CLASS: 10

AVERAGE STUDENT EXPENDITURE: $ (Only in-state students accepted)

M.D.-Ph.D.:   Yes—anatomy, biochemistry, endocrinology, genetics, immunology, microbiology, pathology, pharmacology, and physiology

NBME **Part I:**   Students must record a score.

NBME **Part II:**   Students must record a score.

PHYSICAL ENVIRONMENT

The University of Massachusetts Medical School (UMMS) looks austere and a bit foreboding from the outside. The school has no campus, but there is a weight room (free weights only) and locker rooms. UMMS students can use the pool, as well as the basketball courts, at a nearby community college free of charge. The school has an excellent library that has plenty of space and good labs that are very modern. Worcester itself has a fine art museum.

The area surrounding the school is relatively safe. Many students share "triple decker" housing, of which Worcester has many. The average cost for a one-bedroom apartment is $350 per month. There are no dorms, but there is one very inexpensive government-subsidized housing complex, which has a two-year waiting list.

There are several hospital sites, including the University of Massachussetts Medical Center, which is very new. Worcester Memorial Hospital, St. Vincent Hospital, and Worcester City Hospital are good older facilities also located in Worcester. Berkshire Medical Center in Pittsfield, Massachusetts, is spoken of highly by students who spend their third- and fourth-year rotations here. Students rotating here get free food and housing. As one woman states, "It's the best deal around!"

ACADEMICS

There is competition for grades at this school. Students strongly recommend taking biochemistry, as well as genetics, immunology, and as many nonscience courses as possible, before attending. Physiology and pharmacology are considered to be among the hardest courses encountered by students. Study methods employed by students include taking notes on readings and getting old exams, because the questions are much the same from year to year.

The faculty are a mixture of "the best and the worst." Certain departments are very research oriented and do not care at all for teaching. Other departments, such as pathology, are excellent and the faculty are very interested in students. The clinical training is generally very strong. There are numerous research opportunities. The University has a Family/Community Medicine Clerkship program during January that students enjoy a great deal. Students have the opportunity to follow a family physician and write a research project on a particular community health problem.

FINANCIAL

With the exception of a few other public schools in the country, UMMS is the least expensive medical school in the United States. Students spend between $8000 and $11,000 per year. The school takes only Massachusett state residents and has a special program whereby two-thirds of tuition is deferred interest-free until after residency. This deferred tuition can currently be paid back by one year of service anywhere in Massachusetts or by monetary payback on the interest-free loan over 10 years. Because of the low cost of attending, most students do not feel the need to work, although the opportunity is available. Most students have summer jobs that cover their living expenses.

SOCIAL LIFE

Enthusiastic is the word to describe students here. UMMS provides its students with a friendly and supportive atmosphere. Students selected the school primarily because of the low cost of attending. The school attracts a highly motivated and intelligent student body. There are many opportunities for socializing outside class, including a barbecue, the Halloween Dance, the Coffee House (where student musicians perform), and the Second Year Class Show.

COMMENTS: One must agree with the student's comments about UMMS—it is a great deal! All Massachusetts residents should certainly consider applying to this school, which is getting more competitive because of the increasing cost of attending private medical schools. This is definitely a school on the move, and the direction is up.

UNIVERSITY OF MICHIGAN
Medical School
1301 Catherine Road   /   Ann Arbor, Michigan 48109-0010

LOCATION: College Town

AGE OF SCHOOL: 138 Years

CONTROL: Public/State

AMCAS **MEMBER:** Yes

CLASS SIZE: 207

PERCENT WOMEN IN CLASS: 33

PERCENT MINORITIES IN CLASS: 20

AVERAGE STUDENT EXPENDITURE: $$(In-state); $$$ (Nonresident)

M.D.-Ph.D.: Yes—anatomy, biochemistry, genetics, microbiology, pharmacology, and physiology

NBME **Part I:** Passing score required for promotion

NBME **Part II:** Passing score required for graduation

PHYSICAL ENVIRONMENT

The University of Michigan Medical School is on the edge of the main campus. The medical school has older teaching facilities for the first two years and a brand new hospital. The campus's athletic facilities are a five-minute walk from the medical school.

There has been a plan to renovate the student congregation area replacing furniture and painting. There are several hospitals affiliated with the school, including the University Hospital or Beaumont Hospital, which is in a suburban location, the VA Hospital, which is next to the University Hospital; and St. Joseph Mercy Hospital, which is in the Ann Arbor area and has a great deal of Michigan faculty. The Henry Ford Hospital is termed the "guns and knife" facility and treats many indigent patients. The full spectrum of SES patients is covered by the combination of these facilities.

Michigan Medical School is situated in a college town that has many cultural offerings, such as a symphony orchestra, plays, and museums. The area surrounding the hospital is, for the most part, considered to be safe.

Finding housing does not appear to pose a problem. Housing is relatively expensive. A one-bedroom apartment costs about $400 per month, and graduate student dormitories are about $1900 for nine months. Most students share apartments.

ACADEMICS

One student describes Michigan's work in comparison to undergraduate courses: "It's like studying for a final exam almost every day." Biochemistry and embryology are highly recommended courses for premeds to have under their belts before entering Michigan. Competition for good grades is "moderate" and is elevated by a "gunner minority."

Student-faculty relationships are fairly good, and there are many opportunities for summer research or clinical externships. Students spend about five hours per day studying for their courses. Several students selected Michigan for its excellent academic reputation and the fact that there is a new hospital.

FINANCIAL

The school year will cost the average single student about $22,000. Loans are used by almost all students, and the school has a fairly good financial aid program for students in need of funds. Students cannot imagine working while attending this school. As one student phrases it, "The extra income seems like a drop in the bucket to me."

SOCIAL LIFE

Students at this school feel that they have little time for a social life. There are many school-sponsored activities, such as happy hours, dances, and hay rides, but the attendance is poor.

COMMENTS: The University of Michigan Medical School is an excellent value for in-staters and nonresidents because of its facilities and its outstanding faculty members, who are concerned with both conveying their material and making certain their students have thoroughly understood what has been taught. Students at this school are driven—by their work, by their quest for outstanding achievement, and by themselves.

UNIVERSITY OF MISSOURI/COLUMBIA
School of Medicine
One Hospital Drive   /   Columbia, Missouri 65212

LOCATION: Medium-Sized Town

AGE OF SCHOOL: 147 Years

CONTROL: Public/State

AMCAS **MEMBER:** Yes

CLASS SIZE: 107

PERCENT WOMEN IN CLASS: 33

PERCENT MINORITIES IN CLASS: 5

AVERAGE STUDENT EXPENDITURE: $ (In-state); $$ (Nonresident)

M.D.-Ph.D.: Yes—anatomy, biochemistry, microbiology, pathology, pharmacology, and physiology

NBME **Part I:** Passing score required for promotion

NBME **Part II:** Passing score required for graduation

PHYSICAL ENVIRONMENT

"Columbia, Missouri is a growing town where people still say hello when passing each other on the street." This comfortable and laid-back atmosphere is reflected in the medical school's environs. The medical school is located on the University of Missouri/Columbia main campus. Part of the complex is older, but with the new library and new main entrance, the school looks very modern. The new library has excellent facilities, and students praise it for being so comfortable. The anatomy lab is relatively new, but some of the lecture halls could use renovation.

The University Hospital is currently being renovated and has very good facilities. Students also rotate out of a VA hospital ("fair condition") and Mid-Missouri Mental Health Center. Students find that they see patients from varied backgrounds and a wide spectrum of cases.

The medical school is close to a gym, a swimming pool, tennis courts, racquetball courts, a fitness trail, and a stadium. It is a 10-minute walk to most activities. The school is located in a college town. It is not difficult to get housing. The cost is not expensive when compared to Manhattan or Boston, with apartments ranging from $320 to $350 per month. There is a graduate/professsional student dormitory that is less expensive than apartments and married student housing for $160 per month. Most students live in apartments.

ACADEMICS

This school employs a "traditional" approach to medical education, with the first year predominantly basic sciences and Introduction to Clinical Medicine, as well as Behavioral Sciences and Perspectives in Medicine. Students learn how to perform H&Ps (Histories & Physicals) the second year and take further advanced basic sciences. The remaining two years are occupied with clinical rotations. University of Missouri/Columbia medical students recommend taking biochemistry, physiology, and speed reading before entering.

Competition for good grades (Honors/Pass/Fail) is present but not overwhelming. Students feel that there are ample opportunities for research and regard their faculty as very good medical educators. There are good opportunities for participation in small community medicine at this school.

FINANCIAL

This school will cost residents approximately $14,000, and nonresidents about $17,000. Most students find that it is very difficult, if not impossible, to get by without loans. There are limited work opportunities, and students find that they have time for part-time employment after the first year.

SOCIAL LIFE

There is an active social life at the school, including several parties (particularly in the beginning of the year) and student get-togethers. Students describe their classmates as warm, self-motivated, and ambitious.

COMMENTS: Universtiy of Missouri/Columbia offers its students very good clinical facilities, a highly respected   faculty, and good research opportunities.

UNIVERSITY OF NEVADA
School of Medicine
Reno, Nevada 89557

LOCATION: Edge Of City Limits/Big City

AGE OF SCHOOL: 19 Years

CONTROL: Public/State

AMCAS **MEMBER:**   Yes

CLASS SIZE: 48

PERCENT WOMEN IN CLASS: 30

PERCENT MINORITIES IN CLASS: 5

AVERAGE STUDENT EXPENDITURE: $ (In-state); $$ (Nonresident)

M.D.-Ph.D.:   Yes—anatomy, cell biology, pharmacology, and physiology

NBME **Part I:**   Passing score required for promotion

NBME **Part II:**   Passing score required for graduation

PHYSICAL ENVIRONMENT

The University of Nevada School of Medicine has a great location. The school sits above Reno, affording its students a view of the mountains and the city below. The basic sciences years (first and second) are spent in very nice, newer buildings on a complex just north of the main campus. The labs are new, as are all the buildings for the basic sciences. There is a brand-new family and community medicine center across the parking lot that was built this year by private donations. It would be beneficial to have a car the first year, but it is not absolutely necessary.

The majority of the clinical exposure and most of the third year are spent in the Reno VA Hospital. The patients are generally elderly men and are not representative of the general population. However, this situation is changing, for more time is being spent at Washoe Medical Center, which is a large private hospital. There are a few residency programs, including general surgery, internal medicine, OB/GYN, and family medicine. Students must travel to Las Vegas to do their OB/GYN internship.

There is no graduate student housing, and there are few apartments for married couples. Reno is, in general, a high-rent community. The average cost for a one-bedroom apartment is from $310 to $400 per month. Housing is not hard to find near the campus. The school is located in a relatively safe area. The medical school is about ½ mile away from the main campus, and the medical buildings are very close to the gym and the football field.

ACADEMICS

Students at this school recommend taking biochemistry, psychology, and statistics before attending medical school. Grades are important to students, but they are competing against the curve and not each other. Medicine, biochemistry, and physiology are the hardest courses encountered by students. It is advised that students do not attempt to cram before a test. Continual assimilation of material works better.

The class is very small (48 students), allowing students to know their professors, many of them by first name. One of the strongest points of this school is its emphasis on individual attention. Professors are always willing to listen to students' input and problems with material. There are many opportunities for research in both clinical and basic sciences.

FINANCIAL

The University of Nevada medical school runs about $14,000 for residents and $20,000 for nonresidents per year. In the words of one student, "You learn to live on less money than your non-medical school friends." Most students incur a $20,000 GSL debt in addition to other loans. The school offers both scholarships and work opportunities in the school and the community. However, students do not believe you can depend on a steady job while enrolled at this school.

SOCIAL LIFE

Attending medical school in Reno, Nevada, is an interesting experience because of the numerous nightclubs in town. Some students call it a "nighttime playground," which is nice to have after a long hard day of work. Outside activities are encouraged by the staff, and the students are able to participate in all undergraduate functions. The school has a Christmas Party, a Pathology Party, and Family Day, as well as picnics and parties. Students here are concerned and warm people who study hard and play hard. Most of all, students care about what they are doing and have a mature attitude toward their eduction.

COMMENTS: University of Nevada School of Medicine is a strong school with a fine faculty and staff and caring students. The cost is reasonable and the class size is ideal for individual attention.

UNIVERSITY OF NORTH CAROLINA
School of Medicine
Chapel Hill, North Carolina 27514

LOCATION: College Town

AGE OF SCHOOL: 109 Years

CONTROL: Public/State

AMCAS **MEMBER:**   Yes

CLASS SIZE: 160

PERCENT WOMEN IN CLASS: 38

PERCENT MINORITIES IN CLASS: 20

AVERAGE STUDENT EXPENDITURE: $ (Both in-state and nonresident)

M.D.-Ph.D.: Yes—anatomy, biochemistry, biomedical engineering, genetics, mathematics, microbiology, pathology, pharmacology, physiology, neurobiology, toxicology, and in certain behavioral sciences; also, M.D.-J.D. and M.D.-Masters of Public Health (M.P.H.) also available

NBME **Part I:** Student must record a score.

NBME **Part II:** Student must record a score.

PHYSICAL ENVIRONMENT

The University of North Carolina (UNC) School of Medicine is housed in the medical center, which is close to the undergraduate campus. Students find the basic sciences classrooms and laboratories to be in "fine shape." UNC has an efficient and convenient shuttle-bus system. Main campus facilities are within a 5- to 10-minute walk. The gym is also very close to the school. Parking is a big problem for both students and faculty.

UNC has very good clinical facilities, including North Carolina Memorial Hospital, which contains the Anderson Pavilion, a recently opened critical care facility, an outstanding burn center, the Comprehensive Hemophilia Center, and a dialysis center. This school has made the effort to ensure that its students are exposed to a wide variety of health care delivery systems, including ambulatory care/outpatient centers, HMOs, a student-run clinic, and family-oriented health care facilities. UNC medical students are exposed to a wide variety of patients and cases through the course of their rotations.

The city is in the midst of a housing boom. One year ago it was more difficult than now to find housing. However, housing and living costs are among the highest in the state. An average one-bedroom apartment costs about $450 per month. Most students choose to live in apartments rather than in on-campus housing.

ACADEMICS

UNC has recently instituted a new curriculum that is in keeping with the GPEP report. Under this program students have more flexibility and freedom for individual study and small-group learning. Students generally have two free afternoons per week. Students strongly recommend having a solid background in biochemistry, some familiarity with human anatomy, and a few courses in communications (both written and oral) before entering this school.

The first year is devoted primarily to the basic sciences, and students have their first experience with patients during this year in Introduction to Medicine. The second year provides an organ-system approach as well as further clinical courses, including the Transition Course, which serves as a "bridge" between the second and third years. The third year consists of required clinical clerkships, and the fourth year is primarily clinical electives.

Students find the faculty to be "outstanding" and "interested in what the students think." Research opportunities, such as summer programs and elective courses, are excellent and are strongly encouraged by the school. Competition for grades (grading system: Honors/Pass/Fail) is somewhat stronger during the first semester of the first year and "dies down quickly thereafter."

FINANCIAL

Regardless of state residency, UNC is an excellent educational value. The total cost for first year students is $10,000 for residents and $13,000 for nonresidents. Most students take out loans, with very few students taking out HEAL loans, during their four years at this school. Students find that although it is somewhat difficult, it is possible to work part-time while attending this school. There are several job opportunities in the area of the school, including several medically related jobs.

SOCIAL LIFE

UNC offers its students excellent opportunities for social interaction outside the classroom. There are both school- and student-organized parties, along with other social get-togethers throughout the year. The class is highly motivated, articulate, and, above all, concerned with helping each other and becoming competent physicians.

COMMENTS: This medical school has an excellent administration that has taken steps to "keep pace" with the latest trends in medicine with a variety of health care delivery systems, a new curriculum allowing for more flexibility and less emphasis on rote learning, and a very strong faculty who are actively involved in research. UNC is certainly a fine medical school for all applicants to consider, regardless of their state residency.

UNIVERSITY OF NORTH DAKOTA
School of Medicine
Grand Forks, North Dakota 58202

LOCATION: Medium-Sized City

AGE OF SCHOOL: 83 Years

CONTROL: Public/State

AMCAS **MEMBER:** No

CLASS SIZE: 55

PERCENT WOMEN IN CLASS: 35

PERCENT MINORITIES IN CLASS: 13

AVERAGE STUDENT EXPENDITURE: $(In-state); $$(Nonresident)

M.D.-Ph.D.: Yes—anatomy, biochemistry, microbiology, pharmacology, and physiology

NBME **Part I:** Passing score required for promotion

NBME **Part II:** Passing score required for graduation

PHYSICAL ENVIRONMENT

The medical school buildings are among the older structures on the University of North Dakota campus. Facilities and laboratories are well kept, but students feel that the equipment is not of the latest technology. The medical sciences buildings neighbor the student union and are within easy walking distance of the athletic/sports centers, which have a new gym, racquetball courts, and a pool, all free to students.

The area around the school is relatively safe, and having a car is not necessary during the first two years. However, because the third and fourth years involve a great deal of commuting to hospitals, having a car is strongly recommended during these years. The United Hospital (University Hospital) is a modern facility next to a medical rehabilitation center that is a leader in the field of rehabilitation. Third- and fourth-year rotation sites are chosen by lottery, and several facilities are located in rural areas.

There are several housing accommodations available to students, including apartments, shared houses, dormitories and married student housing. It is recommended that prospective students contact the university housing office well in advance of their proposed admission date. The average cost of a one-bedroom apartment is about $200 per month.

ACADEMICS

Students recommend taking several liberal arts classes, including courses in communications and computers, and medical terminology before attending. Competition for grades has been alleviated by dispensing with a letter system of grading. Courses are graded Satisfactory (Pass)/Unsatisfactory (Fail)/Honors. Histology, biochemistry, and physiology are among the hardest basic sciences encountered by students.

Although other specialties are not discouraged, North Dakota medical school places a strong emphasis on the development of family practice physicians. The small class size provides a very nice student-faculty ratio, which is reflected in the students' favorable remarks about the faculty: "Some of the best teachers I have ever had . . . very concerned about students. . . . They like to teach, making notetaking and lectures worthwhile." Although there are opportunities for research, most students feel that there is not enough time for research except in the M.D.-Ph.D. program.

FINANCIAL

Tuition has recently been doubled for incoming freshmen at University of North Dakota medical school. The cost for a year has risen to about $15,000 for residents and $20,000 for nonresidents. Loans are considered a must for students, and there are several opportunities for obtaining grants, waivers, and low-interest loans. Working while attending medical school is strongly discouraged by the administration. However, there are a few work/study positions available.

SOCIAL LIFE

There are many social events of both a formal and informal nature scheduled for students. The average age of students is between 26 and 27. Several students in the class are married, and students are from a variety of fields, including social workers, biologists, nurses, med-techs, and Ph.D.'s. One woman finds her classmates " . . .

determined, working invididuals who are more than willing to help each other."

COMMENTS: North Dakota has good clinical facilities, an excellent faculty, and strong research opportunities.

UNIVERSITY OF PENNSYLVANIA
School of Medicine
36th and Hamilton Walk / Philadelphia, Pennsylvania 19104

LOCATION: Urban/Big City

AGE OF SCHOOL: 223 Years

CONTROL: Private

AMCAS **MEMBER:** Yes

CLASS SIZE: 150

PERCENT WOMEN IN CLASS: 40

PERCENT MINORITIES IN CLASS: 10

AVERAGE STUDENT EXPENDITURE: $$$$ (Both in-state and nonresident)

M.D.-Ph.D.: Yes—available in conjunction with all basic sciences and several social sciences

NBME **Part I:** Passing score required for graduation

NBME **Part II:** Passing score required for graduation

PHYSICAL ENVIRONMENT

The University of Pennsylvania is the oldest medical school in the nation. In its older, ivy-covered buildings and in the other newer buildings in the complex are modern facilities. The medical buildings are located on the undergraduate campus, providing students easy access to numerous athletic/entertainment facilities.

Classroom facilities are outstanding, with labs, classrooms, and lecture halls having new and renovated equipment. The School of Medicine is in the middle of a large city, yet it has both a suburban and city flavor. Having a car would be nice, but it is not necessary because Philadelphia is easily accessible by public transportation or a

10-minute walk downtown. The cost for a one-bedroom .
is between $250 and $300 per month. The closer you are to
the more money you will pay for housing.

This school is renowned for its excellent clinical facilitie.   ..e
Hospital of the University of Pennsylvania (HUP) is "state of the
art," with excellent ancillary staff and elaborate research facilities.
There are also the Children's Hospital of Philadephia, the oldest pediatric hospital in the United States; the VA Hospital of Philadelphia;
Pennsylvania Hospital; the Scheie Eye Institute, one of the most
comprehensive eye care facilities in the country; the Fox Chase Cancer Center; and numerous other affiliated hospitals. Students here
find that they are exposed to patients from many different backgrounds, many types of medical problems, and different health care
delivery systems.

ACADEMICS

Students here believe that it is your attitude that is most important
when approaching courses. In keeping with the fact that their school
has recently dropped premedical requirements, students recommend
"enjoying yourself" in college. Take what you are genuinely interested in. Not what will "look good." The material is slightly more
difficult than undergraduate material due to the speed of its presentation. Although there is no overt competition for grades, there is a
small group of students who choose to be intense. The large majority of students are relaxed and simply "aim to pass."

Students recommend being organized and not getting behind in
any of your courses in order to do well. The faculty are known
throughout the country, if not the world, and are easily accessible
and interested in teaching. There are numerous opportunities for
research in both the labs and the hospital for interested students.

FINANCIAL

A conservative estimate of the average single student's expenditures
for the year is about $30,000, regardless of residency. Many research
jobs are available both during the year and over the summer. Loans
are available and are mandatory for most students.

SOCIAL LIFE

The University of Pennsylvania medical school is certainly not with-out a social life. There is one "big party" per month plus a variety of faculty-student mixers and coffee houses, dramatic shows, trips to Atlantic City, Night Cruises, happy hours, and theme parties. Students chose this school primarily because of its reputation as one of the premier medical schools in the nation and the diverse group of students it has attracted over the years, from a Vietnamese refugee to a Massachusetts Institute of Technology Ph.D.

COMMENTS: In the words of one student, "Penn is designed to accommodate anyone and turn that anyone into a knowledgeable, caring, and inquisitive physician." Students at this school have outstanding opportunities for basic sciences and clinical learning and the use of the most sophisticated technology available. Another advantage to attending this school is that the student voice is heard and taken into consideration. The relationship between students, faculty members, and the administration is one of trust and mutual respect.

UNIVERSITY OF PITTSBURGH
School of Medicine
Pittsburgh, Pennsylvania 15261

LOCATION: Urban/Big City

AGE OF SCHOOL: 105 Years

CONTROL: Private (With state support)

AMCAS MEMBER: Yes

SIZE OF CLASS: 134

PERCENT WOMEN IN CLASS: 30

PERCENT MINORITIES IN CLASS: 10

AVERAGE STUDENT EXPENDITURE: $$ (In-state); $$$$ (Nonresident)

M.D.-Ph.D.: Yes—available in conjunction with numerous basic sciences and engineering

SPECIAL: Student services offered for disabled students. There are also child-care services available through the university.

NBME **Part I:** Passing score required for promotion

NBME **Part II:** Passing score required for graduation

PHYSICAL ENVIRONMENT

The University of Pittsburgh School of Medicine is housed in Scaife Hall, which students say is "a good basic sciences instructional facility with more than adequate lab space." The Falk Library is considered to be a good place to study, and students are able to use MEDLARS for reference purposes. Computers are available in the library for medical instruction.

This school is well known for its outstanding (and numerous) clinical affiliations, including Pitt's University Health Center, "very efficiently run with good opportunities to see a wide group of patients"; Children's Hospital, is a brand-new facility (opened in 1986) that houses "some of the most modern equipment available"; the Pittsburgh Poison Center; the Transplantation Center; the Eye and Ear Hospital, which houses numerous specialty centers, including one for eating disorders, the Hearing Aid Department, an ophthalmic laser center, a speech pathology division, and the newly opened Eye and Ear Institute; Falk Clinic, an outstanding ambulatory care facility; the Western Psychiatric Institute and Clinic (WPIC), "one of the largest facilities of its kind in the nation"; and the Pittsburgh NMR (Nuclear Magnetic Resonance) Institute.

Students find the area around the medical school to be safe if caution is exercised at night. There is no on-campus housing, but locating suitable accommodations is not difficult with a one-bedroom apartment in the vicinity of the school costing between $250 and $350 per month.

ACADEMICS

"It's only tough at the top." One student says that the competition at Pitt (grading system: Honors/Satisfactory/Unsatisfactory) is only intense at the very top of the class. "The rest of us are happy just passing." Students recommend a strong preparation in biochemistry and a knowledge of human anatomy before attending this school. The first year is occupied primarily with basic sciences. Most students find the second year to be "more relaxed, far more interesting, and somewhat better organized." This year integrates the basic and clinical sciences through small-group learning, problem-solving sessions, and lectures. The third year consists of clinical clerkships, and the fourth year is primarily student elective time.

The faculty are thought of as caring, very well versed in their material, "accessible if some effort is made by the student," and research oriented. There are numerous research opportunities for students, which are encouraged by the faculty and administration. Study groups, taking notes on readings, and mnemonics are recommended as good study methods at this school.

FINANCIAL

The first year at the University of Pittsburgh School of Medicine will cost approximately $19,000 for residents and $26,000 for nonresidents. Students find that loans are "an absolute must." There are work opportunities available, but students strongly advise against working, particularly during the first year, unless "you absolutely cannot get by without the extra money."

SOCIAL LIFE

Students at this school feel that they have time for an adequate social life. The school sponsors some parties, and there are usually several student-organized get-togethers during the year. Pitt has numerous student support services including a commuting student resource center, psychological counseling, child-care facilities, and disabled student services. Most students at this school are Pennsylvania residents; nevertheless, these students are a very diverse group with a wide spectrum of interests.

COMMENTS: Pitt is an outstanding medical school due to its excellent clinical facilities and faculty. This is a school that is interested in acquiring the most technologically advanced medical equipment and in preserving the humanitarian aspects of medical education. The school is actively recruiting minorities and women.

UNIVERSITY OF ROCHESTER
School of Medicine
School of Medicine and Dentistry   /   Rochester, New York 14642

LOCATION: Suburban/Medium-Sized City

AGE OF SCHOOL: 68 Years

CONTROL: Private

AMCAS MEMBER: No

CLASS SIZE: 100

PERCENT WOMEN IN CLASS: 39

PERCENT MINORITIES IN CLASS: 15

AVERAGE STUDENT EXPENDITURE: $$$ (Both in-state and nonresident)

M.D.-Ph.D.: Yes—available in conjunction with all basic sciences

NBME Part I: Optional

NBME Part II: Optional

PHYSICAL ENVIRONMENT

The University of Rochester is housed in modern buildings with a pleasant appearance. The medical school basic sciences instructional and laboratory facilities are fine, and the medical library is currently being renovated. There is some talk of renovating the medical school gym. The new gym would be combined with the physical therapy center in the hospital.

Strong Medical Center is the major clinical facility out of which students rotate ("very good nursing staff, well administered, and excellent and up-to-date equipment"). Rochester is also affiliated with Rochester General Hospital ("a fair facility"), the Genesee Highland Hospital, St. Mary's Hospital, and Monroe Community Hospital. Students feel that they are exposed to a wide variety of cases and patients at these facilities and that they also have the chance to learn the use of the latest scientific technology.

The medical school has its own small gym containing four squash courts, a basketball court, a hydrofitness weight system, and rowing machines. During the nonwinter months, the medical school has six outdoor tennis courts available. The area around the school is considered safe. It is not very difficult to get housing. Approximately one-third of the first-year class live in on-campus housing. Students generally pay from $175 to $250 per month for apartments.

ACADEMICS

One student says that the courses at this school are not hard but are time-consuming. Biochemistry ("it couldn't hurt") is strongly recommended to premeds, along with immunology, genetics, economics ("medicine is a resource which must be allocated"), and liberal arts. Competition dies down by the end of the first semester. Students enjoy the "block system" of learning used at this school. There are three blocks comprising the first year (Gross Structure and Function, Cell Structure and Function, and Adaptive and Regulatory Mechanisms).

It is recommended that students keep up with their work because "work here can snowball fast." The faculty at the school are considered excellent, and students are shocked at how accessible the professors are. Because Rochester is research oriented, there are numerous opportunities for student research and anyone can get a job as a research assistant. Students selected this school based on the quality of the education; Rochester's teaching approach, which is based on the biopsychosocial model of patient care; and the student body, which is "laid-back."

FINANCIAL

It will cost a total of $22,000 for the first year at Rochester, regardless of state residency. Students believe that loans are a "must" at this school. There are job opportunities, but students must seek them out by individual effort. It is possible for highly organized students to work while attending this school.

SOCIAL LIFE

The majority of social events at Rochester are sponsored by students. The class holds large parties called History Meetings, which are for the entire medical center and serves as a way to meet other health professionals/students. Students describe their classmates as social types who are "stuck in their books all night."

COMMENTS: Rochester has many advantages, including an innovative approach to medical education, a very strong faculty, phenomenal research opportunities, good clinical sites, and a very outgoing student body. This is an excellent medical school for applicants to consider.

UNIVERSITY OF SOUTH CAROLINA
School of Medicine
171 Ashley Avenue / Columbia, South Carolina 29208

LOCATION: Suburban/Medium-Sized City

AGE OF SCHOOL: 14 Years

CONTROL: Public/State

AMCAS **MEMBER:**   Yes

CLASS SIZE: 64

PERCENT WOMEN IN CLASS: 22

PERCENT MINORITIES IN CLASS: 8

AVERAGE STUDENT EXPENDITURE: $$ (Both in-state and nonresident)

M.D.-Ph.D.:   No

NBME **Part I:**   Passing score required for promotion

NBME **Part II:**   Passing score required for graduation

PHYSICAL ENVIRONMENT

The medical school is housed in a renovated VA hospital. As a result of this, the architecture is fairly old and interesting on the outside and new and modern on the inside. A car is recommended to get between the main campus and the hospital easily, but it is possible by bike.

There are a variety of hospital sites at South Carolina School of Medicine, including Richland Hospital, which is in excellent condition and houses the Children's Cancer Clinic. The patients at the hospital are from a low SES. The VA hospital has a lot of cirrhosis cases and, of course, veterans. The quality of teaching at this hospital is not as good as at Richland, but there is a lot to be done for those who want a great deal of work experience. Moncrief-Wimmer Hospital is where students learn radiology.

The area around the school is safe. There are many malls and eating places near the school, and students describe the city of Columbia as "up and coming." It is not difficult to locate housing, and there are seven apartment complexes within a one-mile radius and many duplexes across the street. Student housing is not expensive. No student pays more than $200 per month if sharing an apartment or $250 per month if living alone. Apartments are the most common form of housing.

ACADEMICS

Students feel that it is the amount of detail required for courses that makes them much harder than undergraduate courses. Students recommend psychology courses, medical ethics, some phys. ed. courses to encourage fitness during school, and some independent research for summer jobs. Tests are graded fairly. Competition for good grades is present but "masked." Biochemistry, phyisology, and histology are considered to be among the most difficult courses.

It is recommended that students attempt to get "the big picture" in biochemistry. Outside reading and extra study time should be spent on physiology because it is such an important course. The Histology Department is very research oriented. Therefore it is important to have perseverance when studying and, if possible, to get an upperclassman to go over slides with you before the tests.

The faculty is highly thought of, and student-faculty relations are "great." There are many extracurricular activities that both students and faculty participate in together. Anyone who wishes to can participate in research with faculty. Students spend about six to seven hours per day studying.

FINANCIAL

In-state students anticipate spending about $12,000 per year; nonresidents, about $15,000 per year. GSLs are encouraged, and one student calls them "a godsend." Corbett Loans are also easily available but not as appealing because of their higher interest rate. Most students need loans, especially if they are coming right out of college and are self-supporting. Working is not encouraged while attending USC because the school is too test-oriented. Some students tutor for extra pay.

SOCIAL LIFE

South Carolina Medical School Student Association has a Special Events Committee. There are picnics, golf tournaments, oyster roasts, ski trips, and several other activities organized for students. On the whole, students at this school are thrilled that they have chosen it.

COMMENTS: As one woman sums it up, "I believe that our school provides the very traditional education that most teaching hospitals would expect their young physicians to have. At the same time, the school is still in the process of molding its image so that positive change is still very possible."

UNIVERSITY OF SOUTH DAKOTA
School of Medicine
Vermillion, South Dakota 57069

LOCATION: Small City

AGE OF SCHOOL: 81 Years

CONTROL: Public/State

AMCAS **MEMBER:** Yes

CLASS SIZE: 50

PERCENT WOMEN IN CLASS: 25

PERCENT MINORITIES IN CLASS: 2

AVERAGE STUDENT EXPENDITURE: $ (In-state); $$ (Nonresident)

M.D.-Ph.D.: No

NBME **Part I:** Passing score required for graduation

NBME **Part II:** Passing score required for graduation

PHYSICAL ENVIRONMENT

The University of South Dakota School of Medicine is a combination of old and new buildings in which the basic sciences courses are held the first two years. The main building is much older than than the auditorium, the library, and the labs, which are about five years old. The third and fourth years are clinical and most of the hospitals are very modern. The facilities are adequate, and there is talk of expanding the medical school library. The school is research oriented, so they do have technical equipment such as an electron microscope and a plethysmograph; but there is a shortage of study rooms. The school is near the Dakota Dome, which houses a football field, four racquetball courts, four basketball courts, a weight area, a track, and volleyball courts.

Vermillion is a small town, so the shopping, entertainment, and dining in the area surrounding the school are not very good. Because Vermillion is a small city, even off-campus apartments are never more than one or two miles from campus. Housing around the school is not expensive and ranges from $80 per month for a room in a house to $250 per month for a two bedroom apartment. The area near the school is relatively safe.

ACADEMICS

Students consider their work to be about double what they experienced as undergraduates. Most study four or five hours per night. Recommendations for premed courses include an ethics course, shorthand, comparative anatomy, and computer science. Competition for good grades is moderate. The hardest classes encountered are gross anatomy, pathology, and internal medicine.

Students advise memorizing as much material as possible and studying everyday. One woman says, "It seems that whatever method you used in college works here. Just do more of it." The majority of the faculty are helpful and are eager to explain information not understood in lectures. There are opportunities for research especially in the summer between the first and second years. Several of these research opportunities are paid, and students can conduct research in physiology, virology, and biochemistry.

FINANCIAL

The cost for a year at South Dakota medical school is about $13,000 for residents and $20,000 for nonresidents. Almost all students have GSLs. Scholarships are not awarded until the second year. Many students go for HEAL loans; students advise against PLUS loans. About seven students in each class take advantage of military scholarships. Most students say working is not feasible, except for working in the medical school library.

SOCIAL LIFE

There appears to be time to socialize outside class at South Dakota medical school and there are many planned events (some by the Med-Spouses), such as parties, a Christmas Ball, wine and cheese parties, and cookouts. Most of the students are easygoing.

COMMENTS: The small class size and the personal attention given to students make this an excellent school in which to study medicine for four years.

UNIVERSITY OF SOUTH FLORIDA
College of Medicine
12901 North 30th Street   /   Tampa, Florida 33612

LOCATION: Medium-Sized City

AGE OF SCHOOL: 23 Years

CONTROL: Public/State

AMCAS **MEMBER:**   No

CLASS SIZE: 96

PERCENT WOMEN IN CLASS: 28

PERCENT MINORITIES IN CLASS: 2

AVERAGE STUDENT EXPENDITURE: $ (In-state); $$ (Nonresident)

M.D.-Ph.D.:   No

NBME **Part I:**   Students must record a score.

NBME **Part II:**   Optional

PHYSICAL ENVIRONMENT

The medical school buildings are new and modern. The architectural design takes advantage of Florida's outdoor lifestyle, with classrooms opening onto large courtyards. The school sits on the border of the campus, about 1 mile from the student center and 1½ miles from the gym and other athletic facilities. The majority of the facilities are still too new to need renovation. However, there is much construction in progress in conjunction with the new cancer research hospital and psychiatric hospital, which are adjacent to the medical school.

This medical school has outstanding hospital facilities including Tampa General Hospital ("excellent learning opportunities and the hospital is well run"), All Children's Hospital in St. Petersburg, which houses the Children's Bone Marrow Transplant Unit, and James A. Haley Veteran's Hospital. These three facilities are the hospitals out of which most students do their clinical rotations. The Bay Pines Veteran's Administration Medical Center is a newer facility with a strong research program. The Shriner's Hospital for Crippled Children Tampa Unit contains up-to-date equipment for pediatric orthopedics as well as very good research and clinical facilities.

The school is located on the fringe of Tampa, about 20 minutes from downtown. Students say that they enjoy the advantages of a large metropolitan area without living in the middle of it. Tampa is experiencing a housing glut, so housing to fit your budget is easy to find. An average one-bedroom apartment costs between $300 and $350 per month. The area around the school is relatively safe.

ACADEMICS

The first semester includes several "killer courses," as students call them. Among them are neuroanatomy, embryology, histology, and gross anatomy. Biochemistry has been moved to second semester to allow for more emphasis on gross anatomy. Students feel that it is the sheer volume of work that makes budgeting time a difficult task. It is recommended that students take courses similar to those in medical school, such as biochemistry and histology, in order to have some background and a basic familiarity with them before entering this school.

South Florida does not grade on a curve; for example, a 90 is an A. It does not matter how many students receive A's, which alleviates a great deal of the competition among classmates. Physiology and neuroanatomy are considered among the hardest basic sciences encountered by students. "Do not miss classes," advises one man. He adds, "Do a little each day, because the volume of information precludes the simple 'cram' method."

The faculty are very competent and available for extra help. There are many summer research programs that students are encouraged to pursue by faculty and staff. Students find that this school is a "clinician's school," and many chose it because it does have such a strong clinical program.

FINANCIAL

The average in-state student will spend about $15,000 for the year. Most students depend on loans because scholarships are all but non-existent. However, low-interest loans can fill the gap left by a lack of scholarships. The school administration discourages students from holding a job, and many students agree with this policy. However, some students do hold part-time jobs.

SOCIAL LIFE

There are excellent opportunities for interaction with other students outside the class. The student organization sponsors a freshman picnic, a welcoming party, a Halloween party, Med Olympics, and Cadaver Balls. The students here are an interesting group who run the gamut from "beer drinker to ballet watcher."

COMMENTS: South Florida College of Medicine has a strong clinical orientation as well as good faculty and facilities.

UNIVERSITY OF SOUTHERN ALABAMA
College of Medicine
Mobile, Alabama 36688

LOCATION: Suburban
AGE OF SCHOOL: 19 Years
CONTROL: Public/State
AMCAS **MEMBER:** Yes

CLASS SIZE: 65

PERCENT WOMEN IN CLASS: 40

PERCENT MINORITIES IN CLASS: 10

AVERAGE STUDENT EXPENDITURE: $ (In-state); $$ (Nonresident)

M.D.-Ph.D.: Yes—anatomy, biochemistry, microbiology, pharmacology, and physiology

NBME **Part I:** Passing score required for promotion

NBME **Part II:** Passing score required for graduation

PHYSICAL ENVIRONMENT

The University of South Alabama medical school is modern and attractive, but the hospital (for third- and fourth-year clinicals) is unattractive and in a bad part of town. A gym, a student center, a bookstore, and tennis courts are all within walking distance of the medical school. The school is located in a suburban area and is relatively safe. A new on-campus hospital is currently in the early stages of planning.

The University of South Alabama Hospital is located in a poor area and treats a primarily indigent population. Most students do surgery rotations out of this facility. Students also rotate out of several clinics and work with a family practice. The spectrum of patients treated is wide, and students are more than pleased with the opportunities for working with patients in their facilities.

It is not difficult to locate housing near the medical school. A one-bedroom apartment costs about $235 per month. Most students live in and share apartments.

ACADEMICS

"What I am going through now I would not wish on my worst enemy. This is very hard . . . or just requires more studying." These are the words of a first-year student. On the brighter side, students here are not cutthroat and try to help each other when at all possible. Students recommend taking biochemistry, physiology, and psychology before entering.

Gross anatomy is considered to be one of the hardest basic sciences at this school. For doing well, students believe that reviewing transcripts as well as notes is very helpful. The faculty here are, as one student says, "among the best researchers and educators I have ever known." A few "meanies" do exist, but these are definitely in the minority. There are opportunities for student research during summers before and after the first year and during the fourth year.

FINANCIAL

The school year will cost single students about $15,000 for residents and $19,000 for nonresidents. Most students have loans, and several have grants and tuition scholarships. It is possible to work, but students recommend balancing the amount of money earned against lower grades. The majority of students advise against working, especially during the first year.

SOCIAL LIFE

There are social activities for students, including a party after every major exam, formal Christmas parties, charity parties for underprivileged children, and skit nights. The class is a close-knit group because of its size, and everyone knows everyone else.

COMMENTS: South Alabama College of Medicine has the advantages of a small class, which allows for individual attention, a strong faculty, good clinical sites, and very good research opportunities.

UNIVERSITY OF SOUTHERN CALIFORNIA
School of Medicine
2025 Zonal Avenue / Los Angeles, California 90033

LOCATION: Urban/Big City
AGE OF SCHOOL: 103 Years
CONTROL: Private
AMCAS **MEMBER:** Yes
SIZE OF CLASS: 136
PERCENT WOMEN IN CLASS: 30
PERCENT MINORITIES IN CLASS: 5

AVERAGE STUDENT EXPENDITURE: $$$$ (Both in-state and nonresident)

M.D.-Ph.D.: Yes—anatomy, biochemistry, biophysics, cell biology, microbiology, nutrition, pathology, pharmacology, and physiology.

NBME **Part I:** Passing score required for promotion

NBME **Part II:** Students must record a score.

PHYSICAL ENVIRONMENT

Although the University of Southern California (USC) is an older university, the Medical Center consists largely of modern buildings, described as "attractive in a minimalist kind of way," that are about a 15-minute drive from the undergraduate campus. The preclinical facilities in McKibben Hall and the Bishop Building are very good, and students are provided with their own lab bench and desk, a bookcase, and a microscope locker. The area surrounding the school is considered reasonably safe. Students prefer to live in apartments, which average between $300 and $400 per month for a one-bedroom apartment.

Students at this school have ample study space; many prefer Norris Medical Library, which has areas for group studying. USC offers its students outstanding opportunities for clinical training, largely because of its affiliations with a large number of teaching facilities. The L.A. County-USC Medical Center serves as the main teaching center for USC School of Medicine and includes Women's Hospital, Psychiatric Hospital, the Pediatric Pavilion, and General Hospital. The combination of these "separate but connected" hospitals provides students with the opportunity to see a wide variety of cases.

USC also has several other affiliated hospitals that further enhance students' medical education by exposing students to patients from numerous SES backgrounds. The Doheny Eye Hospital is a new facility that has "every imaginable piece of state-of-the-art equipment relating to treatment of the eyes." The Norris Cancer Hospital and Research Institute houses some of the most advanced radiation treatment equipment in the United States, including the most powerful linear accelerator on the West Coast. The Children's Hospital of Los Angeles is among the best centers for pediatric care in the country. Rancho Los Amigos Medical Center, an innovative facility also affiliated with USC, categorizes patients according to their primary medical problem instead of treating them by medical specialty.

ACADEMICS

USC's curriculum is very innovative. Basic sciences are taught by an organ-system approach (normal the first year, abnormal the second year). Students do not find tremendous competition for grades (grading system: Honors/Satisfactory/Unsatisfactory), and there is a community spirit among students. It is strongly recommended that prospective students take biochemistry and be familiar with human anatomy before attending this school.

The faculty are spoken of in glowing terms for their interesting lectures, availability after classes, and understanding of student problems. There are excellent opportunities for student research. "Success in courses is arrived at through careful self-discipline, taking good notes on required readings, and through continual study."

FINANCIAL

USC will cost students approximately $30,000 for their first year, regardless of residency. Almost all students take out loans. There are limited job opportunities, but one student comments, "Why bother, the money you'll make is just a drop in the bucket."

SOCIAL LIFE

There are many social gatherings and parties sponsored by students at USC. There is a tremendous diversity in the class, which is drawn from several geographic locations and backgrounds. Students describe their classmates as open, caring, and very studious.

COMMENTS: The facilities at USC School of Medicine are phenomenal. The access to such an incredible variety of clinical facilities and an outstanding faculty are the school's biggest assets. Despite the steep cost of attending this school, USC is an excellent school for any applicant to consider.

UNIVERSITY OF TENNESSEE
College of Medicine
800 Madison Avenue / Memphis, Tennessee 38163

LOCATION: Urban/Big City

AGE OF THE SCHOOL: 137 Years

CONTROL: Public/State

AMCAS **MEMBER:** No

SIZE OF CLASS: 150

PERCENT WOMEN IN CLASS: 27

PERCENT MINORITIES IN CLASS: 2

AVERAGE STUDENT EXPENDITURE: $ (In-state); $$ (Nonresident)

M.D.-Ph.D.: Yes—anatomy, biochemistry, microbiology, pathology, pharmacology, and physiology; also; special program for impaired students called Aid for the Impaired Medical Student (AIMS)

NBME **Part I:**   Passing score required for promotion

NBME **Part II:**   Passing score required for graduation

PHYSICAL ENVIRONMENT

The University of Tennessee College of Medicine is housed in buildings that are mostly modern, combined with "a touch of antiquity." The General Education Building, where basic sciences are taught for the first two years, is about 10 years old. The anatomy building and laboratories are closer to 50 years old, and there are no plans for renovation of these facilities. One student says, "The basic sciences facilities are all in reasonably good condition." The library is excellent and was built less than two years ago.

There are no fewer than 10 major hospitals within a few blocks of the medical school, which are all "either new, remodelled, or in the process [of being remodelled]." Students say that they are exposed to a wide variety of patients and cases through the course of their rotations. The two major off-campus clinical sites (Chattanooga and Knoxville) provide about a third of the class with an excellent chance to participate and observe health care delivery in a community setting.

Athletic facililties, such as a pool, a gym, racquetball courts, and a weight room, are located right across the street from the General Education Building. The area around the school is "less than safe." According to one student, "Every year there are numerous break-ins into cars on campus and occasional hold-ups of students nearby at night." This very important issue is currently being addressed by both the students and the administration. Finding suitable housing near the school can be a problem. Most students live in garage apartments, apartment complexes, and dorm rooms in the Phi Chi (coed) and AKK fraternities. The cost of a one-bedroom apartment near the school is between $285 and $350 per month.

ACADEMICS

This is a medical school where students are listened to, including in areas of academic concerns. Student committees meet with the department chairmanafter each exam to discuss and eliminate unfair or poorly worded questions. The curriculum is divided into four phases, with the first two phases consisting primarily of basic sciences, which are integrated with influences on human disease. An effort is currently being made to "decompress the first two years." Students find that there is a "smooth transition" between basic and clinical sciences. The third phase is devoted to clinical clerkships, and the final phase is occupied with required clerkships in family medicine and neurology, a course in patient management, and electives.

Students here are enthusiastic about the recent reorganization of their pathology course, which in the past was poorly organized and resulted in a large failure rate on the National Boards for that particular section. Despite the letter grading system used at this school, students find that competition is for the most part "moderate." It is strongly recommended that prospective students take biochemistry as well as numerous humanities courses ("it'll be the last chance you'll be able to take them for a long time to come") before entering this medical school. Study methods employed by students include preparing numerous flash cards and group-studying, with an emphasis on memorization.

According to one student, 90 percent of the teachers consider the students colleagues, while the other 10 percent consider the students objects to belittle and intimidate. However, the administration is 100 percent pro student. There are numerous research opportunities for students, which are both well coordinated and very much encouraged. Students chose this school based on its outstanding clinical reputation as a "hands on" medical school and its inexpensive in-state tuition.

FINANCIAL

The total cost is about $15,000 for residents and $18,000 for nonresidents. Tennesseee provides numerous work/study jobs for students who qualify for financial aid, but one student points out that these jobs pay very low wages ($4 per hour) making it questionable as to whether it is worth the students' time to take these jobs and decrease valuable study time. Students feel it is hard to work the first two years because of the heavy volume of material covered in lectures. The alumni have recently put together a multimillion dollar loan/scholarship fund for Tennessee medical students.

SOCIAL LIFE

Tennessee medical students have very good opportunities for socializing outside the classroom. There are many "theme parties," canoe trips, and picnics sponsored by both students and the school throughout the year. Although most students at this school are from Tennessee, they are from a wide variety of backgrounds and ages, ranging from 21 to 37 years old (first-year class). Tennesssee has many student support groups, including a Big Sibling Program, Faculty/Upperclassman Advisors, Peer Group Counselors, and the AIMS program for impaired medical students.

COMMENTS: One student adds the following comments about this medical school, "The University of Tennessse College of Medicine is one of the best kept secrets in the nation. It is an excellent place to get a medical education. The attitudes of faculty and administration are generally very good. The College is very actively recruiting women and blacks and now would be an excellent time to apply if a member of these minorities or groups." Tennessee has outstanding clinical facilities and is working very hard reorganizing the curriculum, which effort students feel is in the "right direction."

UNIVERSITY OF TEXAS
Medical Branch at Galveston
Galveston, Texas 77550

LOCATION: Urban/Big City

AGE OF SCHOOL: 107 Years (Oldest medical school in Texas)

AMCAS **MEMBER:** No

CLASS SIZE: 200

PERCENT WOMEN IN CLASS: 30

PERCENT MINORITIES IN CLASS: 23

AVERAGE STUDENT EXPENDITURE: $ (In-state); $$ (Nonresident)

M.D.-Ph.D.: Yes—available in conjunction with numerous academic areas

NBME **Part I:** Passing grade required for graduation.

NBME **Part II:** Students must take exam and scores influence final course grades.

PHYSICAL ENVIRONMENT

The University of Texas Medical Branch at Galvestion (UTMB) has the oldest medical school facility west of the Mississippi River. The Ashbel Smith Building (Old Red) houses the anatomy labs and was restored in 1985 to its original (1890s) appearance. Most of the rest of the complex consists of more modern "hospital type" buildings. The lecture amphitheater is equipped with six television monitors on which students may view a closed-circuit demonstration of anatomy prosectioning prior to anatomy lab. Microscopes, audiovisual equipment, and handling facilities for gross specimens are of very high quality.

The medical complex lies within a 10-square block area. An alumni field house has two weight rooms with the latest in Nautilus equipment, an olympic-sized pool, basketball courts, and several other athletic facilities. Immediately surrounding the complex are several residential areas, including an historic district which is listed in the National Registry of Historic Homes Districts. The bay is less than a block from campus.

Locating suitable housing is a problem, as the crime rate is high. However, safe on-campus fraternities offer coed housing at reasonable rates. Rooms in a medical fraternity cost about $240 per month as opposed to $425 per month for one-bedroom apartments. Students agree that it is preferable to live in one of the seven medical fraternities (most of which are coed), but they also note that there are other forms of housing available—such as restored houses, apartments, and condos—and many students live in beach houses near the school.

ACADEMICS

Although the courses are more challenging than undergraduate courses, students do not mind because the material is very interesting. Students recommend taking as many of the following courses as possible before entering: biochemistry, cell biology, embryology, physiology, and microbiology. Says one student, "Unhealthy competition is rare at UTMB. Everyone wants to do well and most [students] want everyone else to do well. There is a lot of comaraderie and working/studying together at this school."

Biochemistry, cell biology, internal medicine, and general surgery are considered among the most challenging courses. One student recommends the following study methods: "(1) attend class, (2) read the textbook, (3) use the note service, (4) flash cards, and (5) old exams." Another recommendation includes looking at old exams and not being overwhelmed by the material. This student emphasizes physical activity. He says, "Mostly, take care of your body! Exercise regularly, eat well, sleep regularly, and keep your hobbies going."

The faculty are very good teachers and many are nationally known. Because of the class size, there is not as much time for one-to-one interaction as some students might want. Research opportunities are both available and highly encouraged, with many students spending the summer after their first year conducting National Institute of Health research for credit with a faculty member as mentor.

FINANCIAL

The average in-state student will spend between $13-$14,000 for the first year at UTMB, with nonresidents spending about $20,000. Most students take out loans, and one of the major ways of saving money is by obtaining less-expensive housing. A few students are able to work in the lab at UTMB or help with patient histories for private physicians, but most students feel that working is difficult until their fourth year.

SOCIAL LIFE

Due to the fraternity system at this school, there is, in the words of one student, "as much socializing available as the student has time for (parties, intramurals, Bible study, etc.)." There are also school-sponsored parties including TGIF parties, a Christmas party, and the all-school dance.

COMMENTS: UTMB at Galveston has very strong clinical facilities, an excellent faculty, and a vibrant and interesting study body.

UNIVERSITY OF TEXAS
Medical School at Houston
6431 Fannin   /   Houston, Texas 77030

LOCATION: Big City

AGE OF SCHOOL: 19 Years

CONTROL: Public/State

AMCAS **MEMBER:**   No

CLASS SIZE: 200

PERCENT WOMEN IN CLASS: 33

PERCENT MINORITIES IN CLASS: 10

AVERAGE STUDENT EXPENDITURE: $ (In-state) $$$ (Nonresident)

M.D.-Ph.D.:   Yes—available in conjunction with numerous academic areas, including most basic sciences

NBME **Part I:**   Students must record a score.

NBME **Part II:**   Optional

PHYSICAL ENVIRONMENT

This newer school is housed in very well-kept buildings in the center of the Texas Medical Center. Universitiy of Texas (UT) Medical School at Houston is interested in providing students with whatever facilities they need, including computers (and computer classes), typewriters, and quiet places to study, as well as in maintaining an attractive facility. There is a gym on campus and a large new recreational facility about two miles away, which has an olympic-sized pool, tennis courts, and indoor racquetball courts.

This medical school is affiliated with several well administered and staffed hospitals including the Shriner's Hospital, Southwest Memorial Hospital, Brackenridge Hospital as well as the Hermann Hospital and M.D. Anderson Hospital. Students at this school are exposed to a large number and wide variety of patients and cases.

It is not difficult to locate housing near the school, and rent is reasonable, with the average one-bedroom apartment costing between $200 and $300 per month. There is an apartment complex available for UT students with a shuttle bus service to and from the school. The area surrounding the school is considered fairly safe.

ACADEMICS

"Everyone is eager for their friends to perform well, and they are willing to help each other out especially when one finds a particular course difficult," says one student about the competition level at this school. The courses themselves are more difficult than undergraduate courses due to the volume of material and the short time given to master it. Students recommend taking humanities such as psychology and histology, biochemistry, and physiology before entering.

Keeping up with the material is recommended in order to succeed. Study partners can quiz you and make certain you understand the material. Students think highly of the faculty, who make great efforts to get to know and help students with the faculty-advisor program and invitations to dinners and parties. There are very good opportunities for research, especially with summer internships.

FINANCIAL

The first year at this school costs $10,000 for residents and $17,000 for nonresidents. Most students find that loans (especially the Texas

GSL) are a necessity. Students strongly advise against working, particularly during the second year.

SOCIAL LIFE

Students at this school lead active social lives and attend numerous social events, such as movies, student organized parties, and picnics. Although the majority of students are from Texas, they have diverse backgrounds and interests.

COMMENTS: UT at Houston offers very good clinical facilities and instruction. This medical school is a phenomenal value for Texas residents.

UNIVERSITY OF UTAH
School of Medicine
50 North Medical Drive / Salt Lake City, Utah 84132

LOCATION: Big City

AGE OF SCHOOL: 83 Years

CONTROL: Public/State

AMCAS **MEMBER:** Yes

CLASS SIZE: 100

PERCENT WOMEN IN CLASS: 20

PERCENT MINORITIES IN CLASS: 3

AVERAGE STUDENT EXPENDITURE: $ (In-state); $$ (Nonresident)

M.D.-Ph.D.: Yes—anatomy, biochemistry, biophysics, microbiology, pathology, pharmacology, and physiology

NBME **Part I:** Students must record a score.

NBME **Part II:** Students must record a score.

PHYSICAL ENVIRONMENT

Most of the University of Utah School of Medicine buildings are new and appear modern. The Medical Center is in a picturesque mountain setting with a golf course in front of it. The old hospital in the Medical Center has been converted to an administration building and is connected to the new hospital, which in time will hook up with a new children's hospital that is currently under construction. The University Hospital serves an indigent population, and its wards are relatively new and modern. The VA Hospital is old but has remodelled all rooms.

Medical students have access to all undergraduate facilities, activities, and classes. The athletic facilities are less than a mile away and include a swimming pool, a gym, a weight room, and racquetball courts. The area around the school is relatively safe.

It is not difficult to find housing within 3 to 10 miles of campus. There are apartment complexes as well as numerous older homes for rent. A one-bedroom apartment costs about $200 per month, and houses generally cost each occupant $300 per month.

ACADEMICS

The courses at Utah medical school are not necessarily more difficult than undergraduate courses, but they are certainly more time-consuming. Students recommend taking biochemistry and histology before attending medical school. Competition for grades is considered very intense, although some feel that this high level of competition is limited to the top members of the class. Physiology is considered to be among the hardest basic sciences.

It is recommended that students compare notes with others and study old tests (a must!). The faculty are caring, and few students have had any problems getting extra help when they need it. There are many opportunities for student research during all four years of school, but the summer programs are better organized, especially the one after the first year. Most students chose the school for its reputation and geographic location.

FINANCIAL

Utah medical school will cost about $12,000 total for in-state single students and $17,000 for nonresidents. Loans are a must in most cases, usually to lessen costs rather than cover all of them. Students feel that working, if at all possible, should be done during the first two years. There are few jobs at the school, but many exist in the community around the school.

SOCIAL LIFE

There are a moderate number of social events for students at Utah medical school. Students generally organize most of their parties, and there is a Christmas Party as well as intramural sports. When asked about the students in his class, one man replied, "The admissions committee likes unique people. We have them."

COMMENTS: Utah School of Medicine has very strong research opportunities, a good faculty, and adequate clinical facilities.

UNIVERSITY OF VERMONT
College of Medicine
Burlington, Vermont 05405

LOCATION: Small City/Rural

AGE OF SCHOOL: 166 Years

CONTROL: Public/State

AMCAS **MEMBER:** Yes

CLASS SIZE: 93

PERCENT WOMEN IN CLASS: 30

PERCENT MINORITIES IN CLASS: 5

AVERAGE STUDENT EXPENDITURE: $$ (In-state); $$$$ (Nonresident)

M.D.-Ph.D.: Yes—anatomy, biochemistry, microbiology, pharmacology, and physiology

NBME **Part I:** Optional

NBME **Part II:** Optional

PHYSICAL ENVIRONMENT

University of Vermont College of Medicine is on a beautiful older campus. The building is homey looking outside and very comfortable inside and is built around a courtyard. The school is safe, and limited athletic facilities are available.

Vermont uses several hospitals, such as Medical Center Hospital of Vermont (MCHV), which is a private hospital. MCHV has just built a new wing. The hospital is slightly understaffed. Maine Medical is in Portland and has both private and public patients. Fanny Allen Hospital is a small facility located in a rural area. The hospital is run by nuns and is immaculate inside.

The school is situated in a small but cosmopolitan city surrounded by lakes and mountains. It is easy to find housing near the school, but it is slightly more expensive than you might expect in an area this rural, with single apartments ranging from $350 per month to $400 per month. Apartments are the most common form of housing.

ACADEMICS

Competition for good grades (grading system: Honors/Pass/Fail) is very intense at this school. Students recommend taking anything interesting and complex that stimulates thoughtful creativity before entering medical school. As in many other schools, students believe the key to success is "doing a little bit each day. On the average, students allot four hours a night to studying during the first 1½ years of basic sciences."

The faculty are friendly, accessible, and like to get to know the students. There are many opportunities for research.

FINANCIAL

The cost for in-state students at Vermont medical school is approximately $20,000 a school year, as opposed to almost $30,000 for non-residents.

SOCIAL LIFE

The social life at this school is adequate. There are picnics, parties, and brown-bag lunches. Students are very enthusiatic about their school and the opportunities to interact with the administration. The student voice is definitely heard here. The student body is both diverse and highly motivated, although students are willing to help one another, especially when it comes time to study for exams.

COMMENTS: Vermont College of Medicine is an excellent school for family medicine. The school is not only concerned about minority and women students but also actively recruits them for admission.

UNIVERSITY OF WISCONSIN
Medical School

1300 University Avenue / Madison, Wisconsin 53706

LOCATION: Urban/Medium-Sized City

AGE OF SCHOOL: 81 Years

CONTROL: Public/State

AMCAS **MEMBER:** Yes

CLASS SIZE: 146

PERCENT WOMEN IN CLASS: 37

PERCENT MINORITIES IN CLASS: 5

AVERAGE STUDENT EXPENDITURE: $ (In-state); $$ (Nonresident)

M.D.-Ph.D.: Yes—available in conjunction with numerous academic areas, including basic sciences

NBME **Part I:** Passing score required for promotion

NBME **Part II:** Passing score required for graduation

PHYSICAL ENVIRONMENT

The University of Wisconsin Medical School is located in downtown Madison in the middle of the University of Wisconsin campus. The basic sciences/preclinical building is an older building with a remodelled interior and adequate lab space. The hospital sites are all considered very good. Students are pleased with the proximity of the medical school to the undergraduate campus because of the near-by facilities. Student unions, gyms, the financial aid office, and the registrar's office are all within easy walking of the medical school.

The area around the school is relatively safe. In order to obtain good housing at a reasonable cost, students have to live a mile or two from campus. It is not difficult to locate housing. A single bedroom in a multi-bedroom apartment costs between $200 and $250 per month, and a single apartment costs between $300 and $350 per month. The majority of students live in apartments.

ACADEMICS

"There is far more independent study, a greater number of lectures, more reading, and more frequent testing," says one student in comparing the work load to college. It is recommended that students take humanities in college, along with biochemistry. Most tests are graded fairly, and competition for high grades is not intense. The first year consists of instruction in the basic sciences, while the second year is taught using a systems approach. The last two years are primarily clinical.

Physiological chemistry, medical microbiology, and pharmacology are considered among the hardest courses for students. Students recommend reading materials very well before lectures, reviewing daily, and organizing notes. The faculty are highly thought of, and students feel that they make a sincere effort to make lectures interesting. Research opportunities are numerous, and summer fellowships are very popular among students. There are further chances for research during the fourth year.

FINANCIAL

The average in-state student will spend about $15,000 (nonresidents will spend $18,000) for the first year at the University of Wisconsin Medical School. Most students take out loans. It is hard to work except between the first and second years. Some students take jobs, but the majority do not have the time or reserve energy to work.

SOCIAL LIFE

This school attracts several older students who have taken time off from school. There are many social activities scheduled by both the school and students, including TGIF parties each month, dances with the Allied Health School and Nursing, and all-class medical school picnics and competitions. Students here are somewhat laid-back and down-to-earth and are sincerely concerned for one another.

COMMENTS: The University of Wisconsin is an excellent medical school, with strong clinical sites affording its students exposure to a wide variety of patients, a caring and knowledgeable faculty, and good research opportunities. The school is located in a good area and has easy access to the undergraduate campus and its facilities.

WEST VIRGINIA UNIVERSITY
School of Medicine
Morgantown, West / Virginia 26506

LOCATION: Small City

AGE OF SCHOOL: 86 Years

CONTROL: Public/State

AMCAS **MEMBER:** No

CLASS SIZE: 88

PERCENT WOMEN IN CLASS: 25

PERCENT MINORITIES IN CLASS: 2

AVERAGE STUDENT EXPENDITURE: $ (Both in-state and nonresident)

M.D.-Ph.D.: Yes—anatomy, biochemistry, microbiology, pharmacology, and physiology

NBME **Part I:** Optional

NBME **Part II:** Students must record a score.

PHYSICAL ENVIRONMENT

West Virginia University School of Medicine is on a beautiful campus located on the outskirts of a small city. The hospital is adjacent to the basic sciences building. Inside, the facilities appear older but are kept in very good condition. There are several exterior remodelling projects currently underway at the school. The main campus is downtown, about two miles from the medical schools, and the Coliseum, complete with athletic facilities, is one mile from the Medical Center. The PRT (Personal Rapid Transit monorail) runs from the Medical Center to the downtown campus.

Although there are no plans to change the basic sciences areas, the school's clinical areas will be greatly enhanced by the opening of a new hospital with a trauma center and a cancer center. Morgantown combines some big city aspects with a small town atmosphere. The area surrounding the school is considered to be fairly safe. It can be difficult to find housing near the Medical Center. Housing is fairly inexpensive, with a one-bedroom apartment costing between $200 and $300 per month. Most students live in apartments.

ACADEMICS

Students strongly recommend taking anything to "lighten" the heavy load of medical school. They believe that familiarization with basic sciences courses such as biochemistry, embryology, and histology will help students during the beginning of their medical education. Competition has been alleviated due to a Pass/Fail grading system. However, some competition for grades does exist.

Students find biochemistry to be difficult, especially if they have not taken it as undergraduates, because the instructors assume a knowledge of the course. It is advised that to succeed in courses, you should study every course a little each day as well as discuss problems with instructors as soon as possible. The majority of the faculty are quite good and understand students' problems. There are ample opportunities for research, and students are encouraged to use their summers to this end.

FINANCIAL

West Virginia School of Medicine costs the average single student about $12,000 for residents and $14,000 for nonresidents for the year. In the words of one student, "One must sacrifice different luxuries to lessen the financial burden. Loans are a must for all but those from well-off families." It is possible to work while enrolled here, and students find it does not hurt their academic standing. The school itself offers a few jobs, but there are many to be found elsewhere.

SOCIAL LIFE

There do not appear to be a great number of social events at West Virginia, with the exception of parties held after blocks of exams. There are a mixture of students from many backgrounds, including a few older students.

COMMENTS: The hospital facilities at West Virginia School of Medicine provide students with exposure to a wide variety of patients and cases. The faculty at this school are quite good, and there are numerous research opportunities.

WRIGHT STATE UNIVERSITY
School of Medicine
P.O. Box 927 / Dayton, Ohio 45401

LOCATION: Small City

AGE OF SCHOOL: 15 Years

CONTROL: Public/State

AMCAS **MEMBER:** Yes

CLASS SIZE: 90

PERCENT WOMEN IN CLASS: 40

PERCENT MINORITIES IN CLASS: 10

AVERAGE STUDENT EXPENDITURE: $$ (Both in-state and nonresident)

M.D.-Ph.D.: No

NBME **Part I:** Passing score required for promotion

NBME **Part II:** Passing score required for graduation

PHYSICAL ENVIRONMENT

Wright State University School of Medicine is a new school that is housed in modern facilities. The medical school building is at the heart of the Wright State University campus and is near every main campus building, including several athletic facilities both above- and underground, for use on rainy and cold days.

The medical science building is very new and has a spacious and comfortable lecture hall. Although the building is new, there are frequent renovations to meet the changing needs of this young school. Because the school utilizes community and government hospitals, the clinical facilities range from the most avant-garde available in Dayton to the VA Hospital, which is not considered up-to-date.

The school is situated in an eastern suburban area of Dayton, Ohio (Fairborn), near Wright Patterson Air Force Base. The campus is eight miles from Dayton and is within easy reach of major state routes and interstate highways. It is not difficult to locate suitable housing in the area of the medical school. Most students share apartments, which are very reasonably priced. The cost of student housing depends on its closeness to the campus, ranging from $200 to $350 per month. A car is considered a necessity at this school. There do not appear to be problems with safety for students.

ACADEMICS

Students find that courses at Wright State medical school cover much more material in less time than did their undergraduate courses. Much emphasis is placed on self-learning. Students recommend that prospective students take biochemistry as well as histology, if possible. Also recommended are computer courses.

There is competition for grades at Wright State. Many students feel that this competition arises from the fact that they are graded by letters (A/B/C/D/F) and are ranked. However, the competition is not "cutthroat," and in general most students are supportive of one another.

Group study and visual aids, together with small-group discussions after reviewing the material individually, will help students do well at this school. In general, the faculty are very receptive to students and attempt to interact with them as much as possible. There are numerous opportunities for student research, and each year a manual is published listing research opportunities. Students are encouraged, especially during the first and second years to participate in research projects in biochemistry and cancer at the Hipple Cancer Research Foundation. Wright State is an excellent school particularly for those individuals interested in careers in primary care medicine. The school emphasizes a humanitarian approach to treating patients.

FINANCIAL

Students anticipate the year to total about $16,000 for residents and $18,000 for nonresidents. Ways of reducing costs include sharing an apartment and living closer to school. The school does not recommend working during medical school but does provide occasional job opportunities that require less than eight hours per week input. It becomes very difficult to work after the second year.

SOCIAL LIFE

There are several opportunities for social interaction outside the classroom sponsored by the medical school in conjunction with the

Medical School Student Council.   Each year there is a Halloween party, a Christmas party, a Spring Fling, a talent show, the Fun Run, baseball and basketball games, a lecture series, the Medicine Ball, and activities planned by each individual class.   Students are very supportive of one another and like each other and work very hard toward their goal of becoming competent physicians.

COMMENTS: Wright State School of Medicine is a new school that is quickly gaining respect because of its excellent faculty, interesting and highly motivated student body, and determination to provide a quality medical education.

YALE UNIVERSITY
School of Medicine
333 Cedar Street   /   New Haven, Connecticut 06510

LOCATION: Urban/Medium-Size City

AGE OF SCHOOL: 178 Years

CONTROL: Private

AMCAS **MEMBER:**   No

SIZE OF CLASS: 103

PERCENT WOMEN IN CLASS: 40

PERCENT MINORITIES IN CLASS: 10

AVERAGE STUDENT EXPENDITURE: $$$ (Both in-state and nonresident)

M.D.-Ph.D.:   Yes—anthropology, biology, cell biology, chemistry, economics, engineering and applied sciences, human genetics, molecular biophysics and biochemistry, pharmacology, physiology, and psychology; also; M.D.-J.D., M.D.-Doctor of Divinity/(D.D.), and M.D.-Masters of Public Health (M.P.H.) available

NBME **Part I:**   *RECENT CHANGE*: Students no longer have to pass each section of the Boards but rather must have a total passing score for promotion.

NBME **Part II:**   Passing score required for graduation

PHYSICAL ENVIRONMENT

Yale School of Medicine is located in an urban area about 15 minutes from the undergraduate campus. The medical school itself has some athletic facilities, but students are able to take advantage of the more complete undergraduate facilities. It should be noted that many of these gyms are run according to undergraduate students' schedules, making it difficult for medical students to find time to use them. There are also several intramural teams for medical students.

The basic sciences classroom and laboratory facilities are very good. The school is located next door to its major affiliated hospital (Yale-New Haven Hospital), and a shuttle bus goes right to the VA Hospital. Students find that Yale-New Haven is an outstanding clinical facility that brings in a wide variety of patients because of its location (indigent population) and because of patient referrals to Yale professors who use the hospital (middle and upper SES patients). There is somewhat more student autonomy in the VA Hospital, but both facilities have an academic atmosphere. Yale also has several affiliated community hospitals in towns such as Bridgeport, Waterbury, and Greenwich. Students are exposed to a wide variety of patients, cases, and health care delivery systems. The administration is also working toward placing more emphasis on medical training in ambulatory care settings.

The area surrounding the medical school is reasonably safe, however, caution is advised at night. There are numerous escort services, and security is considered very good at the school. Many first year students choose to live in Harkness Hall, a student dormitory that costs less than renting but requires students to be on a meal plan (five meals a week), thus making the total cost higher than that of sharing an apartment and buying your own groceries. One man recommends living in Harkness for the first year in order to meet other students. It is difficult to find parking on the campus, and many students take advantage of the Yale Shuttle Bus System (excellent).

ACADEMICS

Yale combines the traditional presentation of the basic sciences with small-group (12 students) learning, and numerous opportunities for student research, which is a requirement for graduation. The Yale System is designed to "foster independent study and decrease inter-student competition," according to Associate Dean Dr. Robert Gifford. A recent academic change at Yale is the introduction of qualifying exams after the completion of each course in lieu of having to pass each section of the National Boards. Students are now required to achieve a total passing grade, rather than a passing grade in each section, for graduation.

Are there grades at Yale? "Anyone who says there are no grades at Yale is absolutely wrong." The clinical clerkships are graded with words such as "Outstanding." If a student does not perform as well as is required, that student will receive "Unsatisfactory" (or its equivalent) and be required to repeat that rotation. This "word system" allows for differing degrees of performance and evaluation.

The basic sciences exams are anonymous and therefore no grades are recorded. However, students who choose to sign the exams may do so and use them as a form of evaluation. Competition among students is practically nonexistent. Students are required to take the qualifying exams (minimum competency exams) after each basic sciences course. Although they are not required to sign the exams, they must seek extra help from faculty or tutors if they do not pass an exam. (Yale has a very strong honors system.) The school has recently instituted a new tutorial system for students.

Students recommend taking biochemistry, as well as several social sciences, before attending this school. The faculty are highly spoken of and considered very accessible after class. A newly added course—Physician's Responsibility taught by Professor Katz, a Yale Law School professor—is being very well received. Yale has about half as many lectures as most United States medical schools; instead, it has many seminars, conferences, and free afternoons for students. Students begin their formal introduction to clinical medicine in a course of the same name that occupies the entire second semester of their second year.

Yale has a reputation as a research-oriented medical school. It is also very strong clinically, and the clinical faculty and facilities are excellent. Each student is required to write a thesis of original research ("not a literature review, but a thesis which asks and attempts to answer a question through student research"). In order to facilitate their research, students are given a stipend of $2000 for the summer after their first year. The opportunities for research are limitless, with students being able to choose from any discipline. One woman is working in conjunction with the Yale Drama School on a thesis that investigates the influence of plagues (including AIDS) on the theater. Yale also has a very active international health committee that sponsors programs in such countries as Africa and England. It is possible for students to use these experiences in conjunction with the required thesis.

FINANCIAL

Yale has an outstanding financial aid office, which makes a concerted effort to address students' monetary needs during the school year. The total cost of attending Yale School of Medicine is about $22,400, regardless of state residency. New Haven is an expensive area for restaurant-goers, but eating at home is fairly inexpensive. Harkness costs about $2090 for nine months plus another $1000 for the required meal plan (only five meals a week). Sharing an apartment is less expensive in the long run (with the cost for a shared apartment averaging $300 per month) because students are not required to be on the meal plan and can save considerable money by buying their own groceries.

The school awards a Unit Loan (which is comprised of the GSL and Perkins loans) to those students who are determined to be financially needy. HEAL loans are a rarity at Yale. Working while in school is not encouraged, but there are medically related job opportunities available in the hospital. It is recommended that students be good consumers and carefully read *all* the information about the loans they are taking out.

SOCIAL LIFE

Yale medical students tend to "hang out" with other graduate students, particularly law students. The classes are very diverse and include several older students. There is a sizable number of students from the Ivy League at this school. However, there are also students from many other colleges and universities. There are several student-organized parties, and students are neither "totally laid-back nor frenetic."

COMMENTS: Yale School of Medicine offers students freedom for research, excellent clinical instruction, opportunities for travel abroad (to learn about health care delivery), and a less intense academic environment than is present at most other medical schools. If you will hear students and administrators agree on one thing about Yale, it will be that it is "one of the least painful ways of learning medicine." By and large, this is one of the top medical schools in the nation.

STUDENT
ACCOUNTS
SECTION

> Nothing in the world can take the place of PERSISTENCE.
> Talent will not; nothing is more common than
> unsuccessful men with talent.
> Genius will not; unrewarded genius is almost a proverb.
> Education will not; the world is full of educated derelicts.
> PERSISTENCE and DETERMINATION alone are Omnipotent.
>
> —CALVIN COOLIDGE

INTRODUCTION

The two major goals of this section are to:

1. Present accounts from minority, women, and nontraditional, as well as traditional, medical and dental students in an attempt to shed some light on some of the problems (and solutions) these individuals and groups have encountered.
2. Provide medical and dental school applicants with a qualitative look at their future education as seen by individuals presently enrolled in medical and dental schools.

The following accounts are a compilation of the thoughts, quotes, letters, questionnaire answers, and interviews (conducted in person and by the phone) granted by medical and dental students across the United States. Due to space limitations, overlapping ideas and comments were either edited or omitted. Those individuals who commented are neither named nor identified with their school in order to ensure their privacy. I am grateful to these outstanding people for their candidness, insight, and sensitivity.

One final note: Headings are sometimes provided to identify a group of students, such as "women." The feelings that are shared are not generalizations but are more specific to individuals within a group. They are not meant to represent the life experiences of every person in the "category".

WOMEN

Sexual harassment and discrimination based on sex were not common problems among most female medical and dental students. The vast majority of women said that being a woman at their school was no different than being a man. One woman added, "Health professionals should not be concerned with gender. They should be concerned with providing quality health care to their patients."

One woman concurred with the above feelings with the following statement:

Being a woman has not affected my medical school experience. Almost one-third of my class are females. I feel the men in my class are able to respect the accomplishments of the women, just as we respect theirs. A problem arises if you let it. If you assert *who* you are and not *what* (female, black, etc.) then fellow classmates will see you and not a classification to stereotype.

Perhaps the discrimination is not overt once women enter medical and dental school, but several women have voiced comments like this one: "As a woman, I have not run into any problems during my training. But, while applying to the school, a few of my interviewers brought up the subject of 'Am I dating?' 'Do I plan to get married and have kids?' I'd be surprised if they asked any of the men these same kinds of questions."

A female dental school student from the Midwest hypothesized that it was the aggressive Northern women who had problems with their male counterparts because they were overly concerned with "proving themselves" as women dental students.

One woman offered her opinion as to the biggest problem faced by female medical and dental students:

The biggest problem is social. There are few women who come straight from undergrad and it's not easy to meet men outside of the medical profession. I was recently dumped by another med student after 3 years because he didn't want to marry a female in medicine. This has happened to 2 other classmates and another recently got divorced because her husband didn't like the demands that medical school placed on her time. So, in spite of the fact that men of the 80s are supposed to be more liberal, I think many of them have ego problems which make things very emotionally uncomfortable for the females who do choose medicine for a career. So, it would probably be wise to include the traditional warning that personal relationships will suffer in spite of efforts to prevent it from happening.

Despite the fact that Southern medical schools have traditionally had a "good ole boy" atmosphere, it is apparent that this is eroding. A third-year medical student states one problem faced by female medical students:

The one area where I have felt some stigma (for lack of a better word) is that pertaining to physical examination of a sexually "awkward" nature. A couple of examples: We've had special small group sessions to learn breast exam techniques on women. No discussion of their importance has been held for men and there have been no small groups for techniques for testicular exams (a comparable procedure with similar emotional stresses). Another incident occurred with my physical diagnosis preceptor. My partner was a male, and although he was allowed to observe and assist all pelvic and rectal exams performed on women (as was I), he alone was allowed to observe and assist with hernia and rectal exams on men. So, now I am in my third year where it will be assumed that I know these procedures without ever having been introduced to such stressful exam situations. To say the least, I'm a bit perturbed at this oversight in my education.

Another female medical student expresses her feelings about medical education in general:

Med school requires many more sacrifices than we (myself and my class) had bargained for. (Before I continue I would like to note that I'm in the top 1/3 of my class and active in a number of organizations so I have not been struggling through school.) Med school requires a big commitment of time, money, and energy. Everything, including most relationships, [has] to be put on a back burner. Although there is free time, most of it is spent with other medical students and there aren't a lot of opportunities to meet other people, except in bars.

You learn to live in a separate, not quite real world, and you realize at age 25 that you've never really had a job or a home. Sometimes, I wonder if I'd do it over. I enjoy medicine, but it's important to remember that this is much more than a job or even a career. If you aren't willing to put all else aside for at least seven years, then med school's not for you.

Another female medical student expressed mild annoyance over certain sexist attitudes of the faculty at her school:

As a woman, I notice a lot of sexist attitudes among the faculty— but these are a minor problem to me. After all, it is still a male-dominated profession so if a physiology professor shows a slide of a bikini-clad woman to describe muscle physiology I'm not that offended. I find the faculty treats me no differently in the important respects like learning course material or test-taking.

However, some women in the class have expressed their dissatisfaction with the above-mentioned attitudes. Someday, when

I am an academic physician, I will show nearly naked men to describe muscle function.

WOMAN/OLDER STUDENT

Individuals above the traditional age range of medical students (22 to 26 years old) have often been told to "rethink their plans." The following is the remarkable story of a woman who began medical school in her mid-thirties and the advice she has to older applicants who are considering applying to medical school.

Being a very nontraditional student, my path to med school was also very nontraditional. The college where I got my B.S. was chosen for maximum distance from my parents so that I could grow without their influence. My major was chosen with a strong intent to help people with emotional disturbances, and with the two choices of psychology or special education, I chose education because for that I did not have to take a foreign language. I took one required science course—Zoology—and got the minimum "C" grade.

After graduation in 1971, I began to teach at a State Hospital in Missouri. I found that I loved the kids, but I did not especially like teaching math and English when I could see that there were many other needs these kids had that were NOT academic.

I met my husband, had a baby, and dropped out of the work force to stay home with my baby and live in a communal situation with several friends. I had another baby and lived in an intentional community for 10 years raising the kids, working on various medical crews (ambulance and birthings)—organized and ran a clinical lab for 80 people, created an alternative elementary school for 40 kids, and generally learned *how to communicate with ALL kinds of people and how to make things happen through my own efforts.*

Four years ago, my husband, my two kids, and [I] left the intentional community to come back to California—kind of a home state for both of us. On the ride back in a Ryder truck with all four of us in the cab for 2000 miles, I decided that if I was going to work as hard as I seemed to be addicted to, I may as well get something tangible out of it all. On the way, I visited an old friend three years younger than me who was in her third year of medical school after having a background in fashion design, and with her encouragement and my husband's support, I decided that if she could hack it, so could I. I had never considered the possibility of myself as a doctor. I had never been encouraged towards that goal and never thought I could do the necessary work until I was 33 years old with many hard efforts already under my belt. At 13 I wanted to be a veterinarian, but was discouraged because "surely I would have to learn Latin for that!"

I enrolled in school as soon as we hit California to begin pre-med which would take me two years minimum. I was told that the first thing to do was prepare for the MCAT for admission. When I added up the time schedule, I realized that if I took all of the required courses and then took the MCAT I would end up sitting out for a year while my application was processed. That would mean I would be over 40 when I got my M.D. I decided to gamble on taking the MCAT early in hopes of getting into med School without that year of waiting. So, I took a review course after general chemistry and sat for the MCAT before any physics or organic chemistry. I did well enough to get an interview at a medical school.

My interview was scheduled for a date after the class was already filled so I was put on a waiting list. Two days before the first day of med school I was accepted. The first quarter of med school was the hardest.

Have a plan of attack and have FAITH in it. Know which schools are interested in nontraditional students and focus your attention on those schools.

I still have a hard time believing that the amount of time a med student puts into studying does not correlate with grades. I study the material because it is interesting and I want to know it and I want to be a knowledgeable doctor. But, the studying and the testing are two very separate processes that are not necessarily related.

My family is both support and obstacle. They remind me of what is real and important when the games of medical school tend to overwhelm. My husband helps me keep my perspective when I take another unfair exam too hard. They continually remind me that I am a valid competent human being.

Unlike my younger classmates, I am not in awe of anyone because of the position they hold. On the other hand, I can set limits for myself and my time. There are times I set aside for my family that school doesn't get no matter what demands are looming. There are times I set [aside] for myself that I jealously guard, and these are the hardest to hold onto. Riding my bike 5 miles to school and 5 miles back is sometimes all I get.

Get your family's support. They are going to be active participants in the process and should be prepared as well as they can be considering no one really knows how it's going to be.

Set sane priorities and keep them. Plan vacations long in advance, and if you have to, spend your financial aid money to get away and be a family again. Remember that a good long-lasting relationship is worth time and effort and will stick by you better than the dean of the medical school will when things get rough.

Be organized to maximize your time and hopefully have some left over for [yourself] and a good movie once in a while.

Collect mentors for good examples. I chose my advisor because that is exactly the kind of physician I am interested in emulating. But, during these years of training, I look to other students for real survival inspiration—the students in the classes ahead of me. They did it, so it must be possible. There are mothers out there doing clerkships and living through it. It must be possible; therefore I can do it too.

Constantly develop your sense of humor—never let it die. Remember—Anything that maintains your compassion and humanity and self-esteem is well worth the time and effort!

Do I regret it? No! Not yet. I'm still hanging in there and there's nothing else I would rather do. The challenges, the constant learning, and the never-ending variety of people who need me keep me interested and willing to jump through the hoops on the way to maximizing my own potential.

REVERSE MINORITY
Being White in a Predominantly Black Medical School

He is one of the only white medical students in a predominantly black medical school. He had a recurring nightmare before he entered the school that all the other students would stop talking and stare at him as he walked into the classroom. This never happened, but he did feel outside the group at times. He says that during class ". . . things are fine, it is during parties when you can really feel left out."

He had worked in a hospital that had many black personnel before entering medical school. But it was his experience with a predominantly black medical school that taught him about black culture. The experience has been "eye-opening," for he had never realized how blacks feel as a minority group in our society.

"We all carry around a lot of cultural baggage. I just don't feel that it's fair that I should be blamed for the discrimination which happened." But it appears that there are other factors that make black medical students wary of their white classmates in predominantly black schools. White students reputedly come to the school and after four years "pick up their degree." As a rule, they are not active in alumni affairs. In this vein, white students at hospital rotations with students from other predominantly white schools tend to be drawn together, away from their black classmates.

His voice is charged with emotion as he speaks about how it felt his first day of school. "I was very scared. But I was determined to go. There was no way they could get me out of medical school even if they shaved my head in the bathroom." None of this occurred and he soon realized that he could work together in the classroom with his fellow students. He feels that he has a modicum of understanding about what blacks must encounter every day because of their minority status. But, as he pointed out, "After I get out of the campus, I return back to a predominantly white society. I can escape. It isn't as easy for blacks or other minority groups."

How does he find his experiences at medical school have changed his attitudes and behaviors? "If I were at a function where people were broken up into groups and someone was left out of a group, I'd ask [him or her] to join mine. Because now I know how it feels to feel left out of a group. I can relate to the loneliness." Looking back, he has no regrets whatsoever about attending his school. He now has a small group of friends in his class who value him for who he is: a fellow medical student and a good friend.

NONSCIENCE MAJOR AS AN UNDERGRADUATE

More and more nonscience majors are being encouraged to apply to dental and medical school. The Mount Sinai School of Medicine has instituted a humanities recruiting program for nonscience major undergraduates, and other dental and medical schools are actively seeking these students as well. The following is an account from a psychology major who is attending medical school. Her opinions are similar to a number of other nonscience majors who are presently attending medical and dental school.

> I am a minority in the sense that I am a psychology major with a liberal arts background. During the first year, my lack of science courses proved to be a disadvantage because many of my colleagues had [had] the courses before. I felt stupid at times, but I still passed everything and still feel my background gives me an edge because I'm more versatile, I am comfortable around patients, and I don't live, eat, and sleep "med school." I encourage nonscience majors to apply and attend.

RACIAL MINORITIES

There has been a slight decrease in the number of minorities apply-ing to medical and dental school, which is thought to be a result of the increasing cost of attending these schools. With few exceptions, every school listed in this book has a minority program and/or strongly encourages applications from minority students.

> I am both a minority (Hispanic) and a woman. I think that both of these things helped me tremendously in being accepted to my dental school. However, both of these things (especially being a woman) have not really been helpful to me as a student. Many times I was accused of getting work "checked off" because I was a woman when in reality I had worked twice as hard as the next guy to get my work done.

* * *

> I am the only black in my class and there is only one other black person in the entire dental school, which puts additional pressure on me. I stick out like a sore thumb. I had to prove myself at first. They would try to use my grades as a yardstick to be measured by, but that's the way it is in any part of American society, so I'm used to that.

* * *

> I am a woman as well as a racial minority. I feel that I had a difficult time here at school in the beginning because of this. I believe that it took a little time for some people in my surroundings to get used to me as well as get to know me and likewise. This pressure as well as that of the course load made dental school quite a challenge in the beginning. As a result of the experience, however, I have learned quite a bit and have matured considerably. I have re-evaluated my perspective about myself, people, and the field of dentistry. My learning experience is a dynamic one in the sense that it is constant and ongoing—a new day, a new experience. As a result, I feel that my character has been strengthened.

VIEWS FROM THE INSIDE
Comments from Medical and Dental Students

Dental Students

> It's [dental school/dentistry] teaching your hands to think for themselves. You sit plastered to a lab chair over a Bunsen burner melting and carving using a stick of wax *after* you've finished studying for your other [basic sciences] classes.

* * *

There's no question in my mind that the best part is actually working with patients and knowing what you're doing in the clinic. It's crucial that you know your stuff when you get into that patient's mouth. The worst part is having the pressure of fulfilling all of your clinical requirements. At times, I have asked my parents and family to "help me out" by being my patients.

* * *

It [dentistry] is a trade, a craft, a profession, and a business. I think you're finding more and more of a concern for business and learning how to run your practice because we're [students and practitioners] realizing now more than ever before that you can be great at working with patients and delivering quality dental care but if you can't balance your budget you'll go broke.

* * *

Praying that your first patient won't ask you how many patients you've treated as you're giving him an injection. You have to have faith in your work and really think you're giving your patient the best you possibly can. But, at the same time, you must learn to work faster and more accurately while learning "on the job."

Medical Students

Having just been made to feel real small by a physician because you made a mistake and then the next minute taking a medical history from a little old lady who looks at you in awe and calls you "Doctor."

* * *

Medicine is still organized as a medieval guild system. The applicant/supplicant must convince the Masters of how talented/worthy they are to become their apprentices. Once accepted, the apprentice's family pays the Masters money for training. And of course, there are various levels of apprentice, the juniormost to the seniormost who is allowed to do many or most things the journeyman does. Having pleased his Masters, the apprentice then graduates to journeyman—who does most of the work and is meagerly compensated. After sufficient service, if he proves himself, he attains Master status. Medicine is the last bastion of such a training system.

* * *

We [medical students] need to be encouraged to be critical in our judgements; thorough in our analysis, creative in our investigation, objective in our analysis, and egalitarian in delivering health care.

We must be challenged to think, not memorize; question, not blindly accept; and learn independently, not passively via lectures. We should learn both the limitations and benefits of computers in education and clinical practice.

* * *

We should NOT be segregated on the basis of grades and class rank whereby one grade point could separate fifty people. It's an arbitrary system driving students to match artificial standards instead of their own. Greater interdisciplinary cooperation must exist among the health professions, nursing, dentistry, social work, physical therapists, occupational therapists, physician assistants, podiatry, osteopathy, and medicine. We must return to the "art" of medicine in contemporary education and improve communication skills.

ISSUES IN DENTAL AND MEDICAL EDUCATION

Acquired Immune Deficiency Syndrome (AIDS)

A Brief Background: Acquired Immune Deficiency Syndrome (AIDS) has not only become a center of media attention and influenced the delivery of health care around the world, but it has had a definite effect on dental and medical students. Currently, most dental schools require the use of gloves while treating patients and many require the use of face masks in addition to gloves when performing treatment that will cause the patient's mouth/gums to bleed. Several teaching hospitals have been designated as AIDS centers. University hospitals and other teaching hospitals across the country are experiencing a large increase in the number of AIDS patients. In 1987, New York, state instituted a new policy among its 13 medical schools: Any faculty member, hospital resident, or *medical student* will be dismissed for refusing to treat AIDS patients. In light of the U.S. Surgeon General C. Everett Coop's prediction that there will probably not be a cure for Acquired Immune Deficiency Syndrome (AIDS) and a vaccination will not be available until the next century, this disease will continue to play a large role in medical and dental education for several years to come.
NOTE: The following are some of the opinions and observations of dental and medical students about the AIDS epidemic and its effect on their education. These accounts do not necessarily reflect the opinions of the AMA, ADA, or other health professional organizations.

Dental Students

Opinions about Treating AIDS Patients

Obviously, the epidemic hasn't had as much effect on the basic science courses (although it is mentioned during the course of several classes such as biochemistry) as it has on our time in the clinic. We wear gloves in the clinic when treating patients and . . . getting our clinical work and requirements completed. You just have so much work to do that it [AIDS] isn't on your mind most of the time. As far as treating AIDS patients, my heart bleeds for the victims of AIDS and their families, but if an AIDS patient needed dental care, short of acute pain, I don't think I would treat him. I know the chances of getting it [the disease] are very low, but the bottom line is there's no cure. If I happen to be one of the unlucky ones who punctures myself through my gloves and somehow gets infected, it's my problem. There still aren't any definite answers about this disease.

*   *   *

It is our responsibility as health professionals to treat AIDS victims. Of course, extreme cautions should be exercised, but the truth is you [dental students] have a much greater chance of catching hepatitis than AIDS from a patient. It's hard not to be emotional about this, but you have to use your mind and do the best you can. If you really don't want to treat AIDS patients, you shouldn't be forced to. But, it is my personal belief that they deserve dental and medical treatment just like any other group of patients.

Medical Student

Experience with AIDS/Terminally Ill Patients

Actually, my first AIDS patient was sort of an unusual case. The guy was a prisoner who was handcuffed to a bed and he had to be uncuffed for me to give my first spinal tap. He was a medium height black man and he was thin and he looked like he was sick. We later found out that he also had meningitis.

It was my fifth week of Medicine [rotation] and I was surprised that I hadn't come across any AIDS patients up until this point. Although it was my first spinal tap and he was an AIDS patient, I wasn't scared. I wasn't forced to do the procedure, I just did it. The door was shut, as is the case with all AIDS patients in order to keep as many germs as possible from entering into the patient's room. There was a guard sitting outside who was reading a newspaper. It's incredible when you think about it, how people in our society are so afraid of AIDS patients. Because they have a wrecked immune system, AIDS patients get sick from illnesses that we would never get sick from. We're more dangerous to them than they are to us.

I've seen some other AIDS patients since that time. Later on, I had this patient who was an intravenous drug user. He had done drugs to "be cool" and be part of the gang. But, he was also very bright and a really nice kid. We had to tell him that he was HIV positive. His reaction was quite normal. He was stunned. We tried to calm him down as best as we could. We told him we would do everything we could do in order to help him.

I've seen other young patients with degenenerative illnesses. I had a sixteen year old patient with leukemia.

Do you feel sorrier or more sympathetic for one patient over the other because of their disease and its "stigma"? When you see someone with an advanced disease it's hard to say, "You screwed yourself up."

An Aside:

I think life is tough for many patients because the physicians and nurses are too busy running tests on them and taking their blood to talk with them. Otherwise they'd be there all day. I think that's part of where medical students fit in.

If I can manage to make them [patients] laugh or feel good by wearing an outrageous tie, I think that's an accomplishment. I had three patients I went to visit after I got back from break. Two of them were terminally ill. When I got back, one of them had died. I wished I had had the chance to say, "Good-bye." Another patient had left and I went to visit him at his home. It was really nice to see him lying peacefully in his bed without any tubes sticking out of him. *Particularly with terminally ill patients who you come to see and know over a period of time, how do you separate your emotions from your education?* I don't take the emotions with me outside of when I am with the patients. I care about them and I think there's definitely an intimacy that exists in medicine that you don't find in too many other places or professions. But, I do not allow myself to become upset. As I said before, if I can manage to make them laugh or feel good when I see them, that's all I can do. But, I think that's a lot.

It is not the critic who counts; not the man who points out how the strong man stumbled or where the doer of deeds could have done better. The credit belongs to the man who is actually in the arena, whose face is marred by dust and sweat and blood; who strives valiantly; who errs and comes short again and again because there is no effort without error and shortcoming; but he who does actually strive to do the deeds; who knows the great enthusiasm, the great devotion; who spends himself in a *worthy cause*; who at best knows in the end the triumph of high achievement and who at worst, if he fails, at least failed while daring greatly, so that his place shall never be with those cold and timid souls who know neither victory nor defeat.

—Theodore Roosevelt